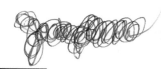

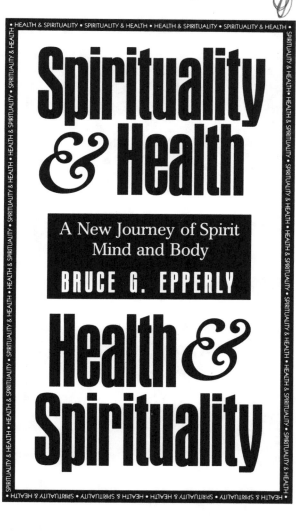

• HEALTH & SPIRITUALITY • SPIRITUALITY & HEALTH • HEALTH & SPIRITUALITY • SPIRITUALITY & HEALTH •

Spirituality & Health

A New Journey of Spirit Mind and Body

BRUCE G. EPPERLY

Health & Spirituality

TWENTY-THIRD PUBLICATIONS
Mystic, CT 06355

Twenty-Third Publications
185 Willow Street
P.O. Box 180
Mystic, CT 06355
(860) 536-2611
800-321-0411

ISBN 0-89622-723-5
Library of Congress Catalog Card Number 97-60029
Printed in the U.S.A.

A WORD OF THANKSGIVING

The health of mind, body, and spirit arises from the dynamic interplay of many interrelated factors. We are all, as the Apostle Paul proclaims, part of "the body of Christ," which nurtures, affirms, and brings life to our ideas and projects. In this spirit of dynamic relatedness, I am thankful to the many persons whose presence and inspiration have brought this book to life. In particular, I am thankful to my wife, Rev. Dr. Katherine Epperly, whose support and confidence made this book possible, and to my son, Matt Epperly, whose life has challenged me to excellence as a parent, mentor, and healer. I have been inspired by Rev. Morton Kelsey's pioneering insights on the interplay of spirituality, healing, and the ministry of Jesus. My theological, medical, and nursing students at Georgetown University as well as the participants in my seminar of "the temple of God" at the Chautauque Institution enabled me to explore the ideas in this book with a diverse and intellectually lively audience. I am especially thankful for the healing spirit in my colleague in the "still point" meditation group and the university healing group, Ms. Mary Jane Pagan.

Neil and Pat Kluepfel and Dan Connors and Deborah McCann at Twenty-Third provided the hospitality of mind, body, and spirit that has brought joy as well as clarity to the process of writing and editing.

Contents

The Temple of God

The Challenge of Health

Martin Luther once stated that "in the midst of life, we are surrounded by death." I had written and taught in the area of death and dying and holistic health for many years, but my academic studies took on a new reality one afternoon in the Spring of 1994. For a few days, I had felt dizzy and fatigued. I assumed these feelings were the result of the high pollen counts that often characterize Potomac springtimes. I gave my condition no further thought until late one afternoon a few days later. As I completed my day's work at the university, I began to feel especially light-headed and nauseated. As a precaution, I stopped at my dentist's on the way home to have my blood pressure taken. When the technician saw the numbers, she counseled me to see a doctor as soon as possible.

By the time I arrived home, I felt worse—I experienced a tingling in my left arm, dizziness, and indigestion. Despite my denial that anything was wrong, my wife insisted that we go to the emergency room at Sibley Hospital in Washington D.C. I felt calm and in control until the admitting nurse rushed me into the emergency room without a moment's hesitation. Within a few minutes, I was hooked up to a cardiac monitor and administered a dose of nitroglycerin. As I looked at the faces of my son Matt and my wife Kate, my mortality loomed before me. I was frightened and, for the first time in my life, I fully realized that eventually I would die and that my usual sense of invulnerability was really an illusion.

After hours of testing, the physician confirmed much to my relief that I had not had a heart attack. But I did have seriously high blood pressure. At first, I was surprised at her diagnosis. I thought I had done everything possible to keep my blood pressure in line and avoid the chronic hypertension that plagued both sides of my family. I regularly exercised and meditated an hour every day. I ate wisely and never smoked. I thought I was invulnerable. I was wrong. Now, I would have to come to terms not only with my high blood pressure but with my own spiritual, emotional, and physical limitations. Though I did not suffer from a terminal illness, I would still have to learn how to find healing in the midst of my own mortality and finitude. This "wake up" call would forever change the way I looked at my life and my health.

That day, I began a new journey of spirit, mind, and body. Although I had spent years studying spirituality and health and regularly lectured on holistic health to medical and nursing students and church groups, I would now have to take my own personal pilgrimage toward health and healing more seriously. I would have to become the embodiment of my own theological beliefs if I were to experience authentic healing in my life.

I suspect that my experience is hardly unique. Health is something we take for granted and mortality is something we constantly deny. When we are healthy, we hardly notice our bodies. We expect them to run effortlessly and quietly, regardless of the quality of our care for them. But, when we have a pain that won't go away or a lump that proves to be cancerous or a "wake up" call such as my own experience, the state of our physical and spiritual health becomes all-important, for illness reminds us that eventually, despite our most concerted efforts at health enhancement, the body will fail us. Discovering our vulnerability challenges us to rethink the meaning of spiritual and physical health and wholeness and find creative ways to respond to the mortality that is our inherent birthright.

Our culture has an obsession with issues of health and disease. Over 10% of America's gross national product relates to health care. Billions of dollars are spent on alternative and complementary medicine, even though many treatments are not covered by health insurance. Health-conscious Americans are bombarded by commercials, television health reports, warning labels, and publications. We are constantly told in the latest diet or exercise manual what we must do, or avoid, in order to live longer, feel better, and stay healthier. Good health, according to the media and the health care gurus, is the result of the right technique or the proper discipline. If we follow the rules—eat healthy, don't smoke, exercise, meditate, and drink moderately—we are promised abundant health. But, as a bumper sticker adds, we will still "die anyway!"

As medical technology becomes more advanced and complicated, there is also a concurrent proliferation of alternative and non-Western forms of medicine and healing. Millions of Americans supplement their visits to the medical doctor with sessions with a chiropractor, acupuncturist, osteopath, herbalist, reiki practitioner, or massage therapist. Nearly everyone is a wellspring of advice on how to prevent illness and encourage wellness. Countless persons, with little or no training, advertise themselves as "healers." Ironically, concern for health has become a new source of stress and anxiety in our time. Where once persons struggled to be justified before God by their good works, participation in the sacraments, and obedience to church teaching, today many persons are hounded by feelings of guilt and failure when they can't get well, don't lose weight, or lack a positive attitude on life. The cost of disappointing the gods of health is a sickly life, loss of self-esteem, and premature death as persons find themselves vacillating between feelings of omnipotence ("I am the master of my health") and impotence ("I am a victim of my genetics, environment, life-style, eating habits").

Recently, many mainstream physicians have entered the arena of preventative and alternative medicine. Their books point out the importance of life-styles that integrate health on the physical, emotional, relational, and spiritual level. Physicians, such as Dean Ornish, Larry Dossey, Deepak Chopra, Andrew Weil, Bernie Siegel, and Carl Simonton, have become media celebrities through their affirmation of the importance of prayer and other spiritual practices in a healthy life. The power of prayer and the "faith factor" are now routinely cited as essential components in a healthy life-style. A growing number of physicians offer to pray with their patients. Studies on the impact of meditation or the "relaxation response" demonstrate that the regular practice of meditation lowers high blood pressure, relieves stress, and enhances creativity.[1] Some of today's physicians sound amazingly like revival preachers in their zeal to proclaim the necessity of imaging, meditation, attitudinal healing, prayer, vegetarian diets, and fiber in securing us both health and happiness. Yet, equally significant is the fact that few of these physicians have had the theological training necessary to understand the spiritual dimensions of health, illness, and unanswered prayer.

Strangely enough, mainstream Christian ministers and theologians have been virtually silent in proposing a Christian vision of spirituality and health.[2] Further, most of the physicians who accent the importance of spirituality for healthful living ground their beliefs in Asian, vaguely new age, or new thought philosophies. Although Christians may gain much from their counsel, they seldom are able to integrate these new insights with their own Christian faith. As they read books on meditation, spiritual healing, yoga, or creative aging, many Christians wonder what these practices have to do with the teachings of Jesus of Nazareth and their own Christian churches. Some even ask themselves if participation in alternative and complementary medical modalities contradicts the teachings of Scripture and loyalty to Christ. Their efforts to understand alternative medicine and preventative health would be strengthened and their health more fully addressed if the practices of holistic health and alternative medicine could be related to the healing message of Christianity.

The goal of this book is simply to provide a Christian vision of health and wellness for contemporary persons. Good health, spiritual healing, alternative medicine, prevention and personal responsibility, and conscious aging and dying all have a place in the Christian vision of reality and are grounded in the Christian vision of healing and wholeness. But Christians must rediscover and reclaim the biblical and spiritual heritage of healing if this synthesis is to be achieved.

CHAPTER ONE

CHRISTIANITY AND HEALTH

Scripture has much to say about health and healing. But much of the scriptural and theological tradition of Christianity remains unexplored, misunderstood, or only superficially studied. In the biblical tradition, our relationship to God is reflected in our life-style—in the areas of diet, vocation, ethical behavior, and in our attitudes toward time, possessions, and illness. From the very beginning of the scriptural witness, the physical body, sexuality, and relationships are defined as "good" (Genesis 1:25–31; 2:21–25). Unnoticed by most readers is the fact that although creation is described as good, it is never called perfect. Only God is perfect and eternal. Aging and death are essential elements in the human adventure and have a place in God's good creation. In the tension between goodness and perfection, we discover the adventure of health and healing and the dynamic presence of God in our lives.

To embrace a creative vision of health and healing today, Christians must rediscover the healing message and practices of the Great Physician. Although nearly one-fifth of the accounts of Jesus' life relate to health issues, few Christians take note of their relevance to persons today. Although some churches, most notably Episcopalian, Roman Catholic, and

Pentecostal, have initiated healing services, many Christians have never heard a sermon on healing and identify Christian healing solely with the histrionic and manipulative antics of televangelists and faith healers, or the random and inscrutable acts of an arbitrary God.

Scripture identifies Jesus as a healer of mind, body, and spirit. Jesus' first public sermon outlined his image of salvation or shalom:

> The Spirit of the Lord is upon me, because he has anointed me to preach good news to the poor. He has sent me to proclaim release to the captives and recovering of sight to the blind, to set at liberty those who are oppressed and to proclaim the acceptable year of the Lord (Luke 4:18–19).

Later, when John the Baptist's disciples ask if Jesus is the Messiah, Jesus responds, "the blind receive their sight, the lame walk, lepers are cleansed, and the deaf hear, the dead are raised up, and the poor have good news preached to them" (Luke 7:22). While both passages lift up the political and ethical aspects of God's reign, recognized today by liberation and feminist theologians as essential to the Gospel message, they also lift up the significance of personal healing as a sign of God's reign in the universe. In the spirit of his Hebraic ancestors, Jesus saw salvation as relating to the totality of human life—physical, emotional, spiritual, environmental, vocational, economic, and political. Indeed, the ministry of Jesus suggests that salvation means health and wholeness in the totality of human existence, in this life as well as beyond the grave.

Today, as physicians such as Larry Dossey explore the power of prayer, faith, and the placebo effect in physical healing, Christians are reminded of Jesus' own words to a woman cured of chronic illness, "your faith has made you well"

(Matthew 9:18–22, Mark 5:24–34; Luke 8:43–48). As creatures created in God's image, we are born with a bias toward health, which is reflected in the primarily automatic workings of the cardiovascular, immune, and nervous systems.

Contrary to many Jews of his time and many Christians and new agers in our time, Jesus proclaimed that illness is not simply a result of divine punishment, God's will, or the inexorable workings of cause and effect or karma. Illness results from a multitude of causes, both spiritual and physical. The God Jesus proclaimed is the God of healing and life and not the source of sickness and death. Health and healing, as reflected both in the workings of our body and the impact of spirituality on personal well-being, are embodiments of God's desire that all persons "might have abundant life" (John 10:10).

Without a doubt the greatest witness to the significance of embodiment and the divine redemption of physical existence in all its forms is the incarnation itself. Christianity is unique among the world religions in its affirmation that divine love must be embodied. The God who "so loved the world that he gave [his] only begotten son" (John 3:16) is revealed in the Word that becomes flesh and dwells among us "full of grace and truth" (John 1:14). In his own care for the sick, dying, and outcast, Jesus revealed the full nature of divine salvation and became, along with Hippocrates, the model for Western medicine. Christians can rejoice that the incarnation is not limited to the life of Jesus, but that God's healing work is revealed in greater and lesser degrees in all things. To paraphrase the language of the early theologians of the church, wherever there is truth *and* healing, Christ is present as its source.

Today's Christians can also take heart in the recent studies on the power of prayer. Larry Dossey and others have shown clearly that prayer makes a difference in health and healing.[1] As I will point out later in this book, spiritual prayer should be a medicinal companion to aspirin, fluids, beta blockers, prozac, and chemotherapy, if we are to address creatively and faithfully the totality our lives. Other studies have noted the value of active participation in religious communities for health and positive aging. As one church notice recommends: "Join us for church Sunday: you'll feel better and live longer!"

While many Christians have scorned physical existence as imperfect and evil or have seen this lifetime as "the front porch of eternity," authentic Christianity affirms that every aspect of human life—body, sexuality, eating, praying, meditating, and serving—may become a means to encounter God. It is natural for Christians to seek good health for themselves and others, both individually and politically. We are, as Psalm 139:14 proclaims, "fearfully and wonderfully made." The divine artist "knit [our bodies] together in our mother's womb" (Psalm 139:13). Even the most cursory reading of the Song of Solomon invites us to celebrate the beauty of our physical bodies, both in terms of their external appearance and their invisible workings.

Authentic piety demands that we give thanks daily for the blessings of physical existence, the gifts of the senses, and the operations of the mind. We must discover not only that the "heavens declare the glory of God," but this same glory is also proclaimed by our immune and cardiovascular systems, the monthly ovarian cycles, the colon and intestines, and the liver and spleen! Medicine can heal precisely because the body, at every level, aims at healing.

Scripture proclaims that the body is the "temple of God" (1 Corinthians 6:19). Paul's admonitions to the Christians at Corinth are grounded in the importance of bodily existence. Intercourse with prostitutes is forbidden not merely because of its impact on the body, but because of its impact on our spiritual, emotional, and relational lives. As the temple of God, the body is the shrine in which the Holy Spirit and the Christ within find their home (1 Corinthians 6:12–20). In the spirit of Paul's words to the Corinthians, we can affirm the sacramental nature of embodiment. Our bodies, like the rainbow and the cross, reflect God's care for all things and God's covenant of healing love. In our spiritual examinations, we must ask ourselves if we are treating our bodies in a sacred manner. Are we, to quote Paul, "glorifying God" with our bodies (1 Corinthians 12:20)? Do our eating, recreation, work style, and behavior reflect a recognition that God is embodied in our own physical lives? Sadly, for most of us, the answer is "no." We often eat ungratefully and unconsciously. Our consumption of food and drink often fails to take into account the "other weight problem," malnutrition in our own land and across the globe. Sadly, we do not respect our bodies. We leave their care to physicians and nurses and maltreat them until they break down.

The biblical tradition asserts that there is another way of life. We are challenged every day to choose life and not death as we glorify God in our bodies. As W.H. Auden counsels in his Christmas play, *For the Time Being*, we are to "love [God] in the world of the flesh."[2] The path to physical and spiritual health is not meant to be one more task necessary for our salvation. We belong to God and stand in God's circle of love whether or not we are physically healthy. God's grace is not based on our own achievements in righteousness, stress reduction, or weight loss. Rather, a fully healthy life-style is grounded in our response to the grace of God revealed in God's ever-present care for our bodies, minds, and spirits. Because God loves our flesh, we are called to love our bodies and the bodies of our neighbors.

A rich young man once asked Jesus, "what must I do to be saved?" Persons today, recognizing that the Greek word for salvation and health is one and the same, often ask, "what must I do to be healthy and whole?" Issues of health and illness are theological and spiritual issues. How we take care of ourselves—body, mind, and spirit—is a matter of faith and unfaith. While faith and spiritual growth do not insure physical well-being (saints die of cancer and drug lords live comfortably into old age), we are challenged, nevertheless, to live our lives and care for our bodies in dynamic relationship to the God of health and salvation. As we will discover, health and illness are ultimately a matter of our spiritual connectedness or disconnectedness to the ground of all health and wholeness.

"You are God's temple and God's spirit dwells in you," writes the apostle Paul (1 Corinthians 3:16). Not only our body, but our being is a shrine of God. God's loving energy and lively spirit course through our veins and intestines, but also through our thoughts, imagination, emotions, and memories. We are both corporately and individually members of "the body of Christ" (1 Corinthians 12), an organism of many gifts and talents, of many aspects and possibilities, each of which must be honored if we are to claim the abundance that is our birthright as God's beloved children.

In speaking of the relationship of ecology and spirituality, Catholic theologian and ecologist Thomas Berry asserts that the universe is the primary word of God. We can equally affirm that our body, minds, and spirits are the most directly experienced revelations of God. When we bring our lives in their totality to God, then the body truly becomes a temple and the spirit a holy place.

As Christians seek to reflect on health and healing, they must remember Paul's admonition, "be not conformed to the world, but be transformed by the renewing of your mind" (Romans 12:2). A Christian vision of spirituality and health—like a Christian ethic and life-style—will be countercultural in many ways. It will affirm the role of spirituality in a technologically obsessed world. It will affirm the body and the practice of medicine as gifts from God. It will accept the reality of death and suffering and challenge those who end life prematurely or maintain life unnecessarily. It will also affirm the spiritual-emotional-physical-relational unity of life and challenge all types of dualism, both spiritual and secular. In the spirit of the universal nature of divine truth and revelation, it will be multicultural in its integration of ancient and modern and east and west. It will seek health and healing, while avoiding the extremes of narcissistic omnipotence and passive impotence.

The vision of our lives as the "temple of God" is grounded in a living and grateful relationship to the Creator of all things in earth and heaven. The German mystic Meister Eckhart once stated that "if the only prayer you make is thank you, that will be enough." Gratitude is the starting point for a life of health and faith: simply by thanking God for the "temple," for the blue sky and the green fields, for the rushing wind and the stormy sea, for the gift of the senses and the ability to love, for the beating heart and the digesting stomach. None of these depend fully on our efforts. They come as graces and ordinary miracles. But we can enhance our experience of embodiment in all its dimensions and we can live abundantly in all the seasons of life by living a life of gratitude and care, that is, by placing God at the center of all our efforts at health and well-being.

Health is a spiritual issue. We glorify and worship God by the care we give to God's creation, the intimate creation of our bodies and spirits, and the ambient creation of the earth and our fellow creatures. In the chapters ahead, I invite you to join me in a sacred journey toward spiritual well-being and physical health. We will explore the frontiers of health and healing as they relate to physical existence, stress, spiritual growth, personal healing, aging, and dying. The book's approach will be intensely practical. Theology, at its best, begins and ends with everyday as well as dramatic experiences of brokenness and healing. In this spirit, I will weave theological reflection and medical research with practical methods of physical, emotional, and spiritual health as these relate to the totality of life. Each particular emphasis ultimately relates to the whole of life, since all aspects of life exist in dynamic relationship. The separation of emotional, physical, spiritual, and relational, or diet, exercise, rest, and prayer, is ultimately artificial, for there is only one world and one God, and our embodiment reflects the multidimensional unity of one whole being. Let us journey together the path of health and healing with God as our guide and companion.

QUESTIONS FOR REFLECTION AND DISCUSSION

1) How do you evaluate your current health condition? What is your image of health and illness?

2) Have you ever experienced a critical or chronic illness of mind or body? How would you describe your experience? Were there any spiritual components to your illness?

3) The New Testament sees Jesus as a healer and miracle worker. How do you understand the healings of the New Testament? Are such healings still possible today?

4) What is your church's attitude toward spiritual and faith healing? Have you ever been to a healing service? What was your response to the service?

5) How do you understand the relationship of spirituality and medicine? Can these two disciplines creatively complement each other?

CHAPTER TWO

CARING FOR THE TEMPLE

I. The Theology of Embodiment

In a recent pictorial book on the human body, scientist and author Lewis Thomas describes the body as an "incredible machine." At first glance the use of the word "machine" elicits the images of mechanistic lifelessness and piecemeal thinking characteristic of modern technology. Yet, Thomas notes that the word "machine" does not have its roots in mechanistic scientific thinking. It arises from the Indo-European word "magh," which is a cognate for "magic." Our bodies are incredibly magical. Psalm 139's description of the body as "fearfully and wonderfully made" captures the awe we experience when we look at the heavens above and then gaze into an electron microscope and marvel at the intricacy and beauty of a recently fertilized egg or the mini-universe of a liver or blood cell. Our bodies are truly magical in their intricacy and interconnectedness!

Christian faith affirms the marvel of embodiment. Although historically some Christians have followed the teachings of Plato's Socrates in the dialogue *Phaedo* and the first-century Gnostics who saw the body as "a prison house," whose demands chain the soul to the earth, the New

Testament church saw the body as a "temple" and shrine for the living God. In contrast to those Corinthians who saw embodiment as a deterrent to spiritual growth or a matter of moral or spiritual indifference, Paul uses the physical body, including its most humble and earthly parts, as the primary metaphor for the "body of Christ," the communion of saints enlivened by the spirit of Christ.

In each generation, those who would flee the body and mortify the flesh are counseled to reflect upon the manger and the cross. Amid the earthiness of childbirth and the blood and sweat of the Cross, Christians discover that the divine plan of salvation occurs through embodiment in all its earthiness from life to death and not in some disembodied idea or spiritual practice.

I noted earlier Thomas Berry's assertion that the universe is the primary, or fundamental, revelation of God. In fact, our most immediate encounter with God occurs in the context of our bodily existence. Apart from the seldom-noticed optic nerves, we could not gaze upon the starry skies and the majestic mountains; we could not hear the sound of a waterfall or a Beethoven symphony or Beatles ballad apart from the intricate workings of the eardrum and auditory nerves. When we observe our bodies, we are indeed observing God's self-revelation in all its variety and uniqueness.

In the spirit of the Pauline metaphor, our embodiment is God's dwelling place in the world of the flesh. Christians today must affirm a theology of embodiment rather than a theology of detachment or world denial. Flesh is not senseless matter or an obstacle to spiritual experience, it is the dwelling place of God and the ultimate ground of spirituality and salvation.

The "temple of God" is dynamic and alive. It encompasses our whole being, including the mind, emotions, and spirituality. As we consider the intricate relationships of thought, feeling, and embodiment, we cannot accurately determine where the body ends and the mind begins. Body permeates the mind, and mind permeates the body. To paraphrase Psalm 139, where shall we go to escape our embodiment? All of our actions, from sexual relations to digestion, are psychosomatic and spiritual in their depths, and the greatest flights of mystical experience are grounded in the unnoticed, but ever-present, workings of the body.

To the surprise of many spiritual seekers, the temporality and ephemeral nature of embodiment are precisely the source of its spiritual significance. Following the Greek philosophers, many early Christians came to believe that the body was evil. They assumed that only the eternal and unchanging realities could participate in the eternity of God. Yet, in their quest for the "god of the philosophers," they neglected the God of Jesus and the Hebraic parents of our faith. In contrast to those who saw change as a fall from perfection, the Hebraic and early Christian traditions saw change at the heart of God's existence. God is active, dynamic, and personal. Although God's promises are "the same yesterday, today, and tomorrow," God's fidelity is personal, relational, and ever-changing. God is always doing a new thing, whether in our spiritual lives or in our bodies. We discover God not by fleeing the world of change, but by immersing ourselves in God's temporality and, thereby, discovering God's will for our lives and our time. A personal relationship with God is always temporal, dynamic, and lively.

Reflecting the wisdom of its Creator, the body reveals the same dynamic movement. In its constant cellular living and dying, the body reflects God's own lively relationship with the world, which includes death and degeneration as the necessary prelude to birth and growth. Further, the body's essential bias toward health and healing incarnates God's own gentle movements of redemption. What Jesus exhibited in the dramatic healings of the sick is just as wonderfully, although less dramatically, revealed in the immune system's protection of the body and the cardiovascular system's role in the healing of injuries. Like the God who fashions it, the body transforms and redeems the materials of life as it seeks abundant life for itself and others.

The wisdom and creativity of God are revealed whether we look at the mountaintops or our fingernails. Take a minute to gaze upon your own face or the face of a loved one. How unique and complex it is. Reflect on the mechanics involved in speaking, walking, or reading this book. Then, explore the many small universes of the body with an electron microscope. Everywhere you look, even at disease cells, there is something magical for those whose vision is attuned to God's wisdom. As William Blake proclaims, "if the doors of perception were cleansed, everything would appear as it is, infinite."[1] If we want to be truly close to God, we must stand in awe of God's embodied revelation. If God is truly omnipresent, then God is constantly being revealed in the movements of our bodies and minds.

Biblical spirituality counsels us to love God in the world of the flesh. We love the world of the flesh, first of all, because it is loved by God. God cares for the earth and for all living things. God counts the hairs on our heads, clothes the grass of the field, and feeds the sparrows. Embodiment in all of its forms, human and nonhuman, is the handiwork of a patient and artistic God who delights in evolving new forms of life from age to age (Proverbs 8).

God delights in the intimacy of sexuality and conception. The call to be "fruitful and multiply" is given to humankind as well as the nonhuman realm. Adam's exclamation as he discovers a partner in life is the foundation of creative love: "This, at last, is bone of my bone and flesh of my flesh" (Genesis 2:23). Adam's exclamation is much more than an anatomy lesson, it is an affirmation that marriage, sexuality, and relationship all reflect the divine creativity in our midst. As we affirm our embodiment, whether we are married, single, or celibate, we follow the example of the first couple who lived together "naked and unashamed" (Genesis 2:25).

Hatred of the body and shame over one's appearance are the result of the sin of cultural stereotypes, sexual abuse and harassment, and unhealthy relational and life-style habits. The biblical account of the Fall suggests that body denial and embarrassment are rooted in humankind's disconnectedness from its loving Creator. As the Song of Songs asserts, the body is meant for appreciation, enjoyment, and intimacy. Even the language of the Old Testament suggests that sexuality is meant to be a way of *knowing* oneself, the other, and God.

Loving God in the flesh is also reflected in the biblical concern for justice. We love the creator by loving the creatures. When Amos proclaims "let justice roll down like waters and righteousness like an everflowing stream," he is asserting the interdependent and psychosomatic nature of human life. Love must be expressed in just and life-affirming actions. Spirituality must be embodied in just social structures that bring health and joy to the bodies and spirits of all persons. In this same spirit, Matthew's Gospel asserts that as we care for the bodies of the least of these, providing food, clothing, water, and comfort, we are also providing sustenance for God. Biblical spirituality knows nothing of the separation of mind and body, or faith and politics, characteristic of the modern era.

Jesus of Nazareth, as the incarnation of God, lived and loved as God in the flesh. Food, drink, celebration, friendship, rest, and touch all figure significantly in the New Testament portrait of Jesus. Jesus is not a world-denying ascetic nor does Jesus scorn his own or anybody else's flesh. The Gospels speak of Jesus admiring and enjoying the birds and flowers, sunshine on the Sea of Galilee, sailing, wedding parties, and the fellowship and touch of friends. Long before the advent of the holistic health movement, Jesus' ministry expressed the unity of body, mind, and spirit. Touching the body comforts the spirit, just as spiritual transformation brings health to the body. Healing of illness enables persons to devote their lives to God and live productive and joyful lives. Healing faith brings new life to the body as well as the spirit.

Anglican Archbishop William Temple once claimed that unless you saw God's presence in the rising sun, you would not be able to find God in the resurrection of the Son of Man. Today, I would add that unless you see God's presence in the transformation of food into energy or the healing of a wound, you will not see God in the saving of a soul! Our bodies are cathedrals and temples—like Notre Dame, Chartres, or Lourdes. Our embodiment is our invitation to seek and find God in the ordinary acts of life. Like other holy places, our bodies should be shrines where we expect to find God, whether in good health or in illness, youth or aging, birthing or dying. But, many of us, as we reflect on our bodily life, must confess that "surely God was in this place but we did not know it."

As we learn to love our bodies, we are challenged to love all other bodies. We love the creator by caring for the creation, be it human or nonhuman. Although philosopher Alfred North Whitehead once stated that "life is robbery," we must learn to caretake for the earth, to go beyond waste and competition, and learn to reverence all of life as a gift and revelation of God, for our health and the health of the earth are intricately connected.

Today, the "sins of the flesh" are not so much those of carnality, but our failure to love fully our own bodies and the bodies of our fellow creatures. Sin is revealed in our neglect of the body. By the passivity of omission or the activity of commission, sins of the flesh wound our bodies and the bodies of others. Today's sins of the flesh are manifest in the "weight problem" that brings cardiovascular disease to the wealthy and starvation to the poor. The sin of disobedience is revealed in our failure to follow the inner laws of embodiment and our lack of respect for our own bodies.

What we eat and drink and our attitude toward life is a matter of faith. When we are alienated from our bodies and their needs, we are like the branches that wither when they are severed from the life-giving and spiritually nurturing energy of the vine (John 15). Christians today are called to love God in the flesh. We are to seek healing in our bodies because the God we worship seeks healing and abundant life for ourselves and all other beings.

As we explore what it means to take care of the temple of God, we will specifically reflect in this chapter on the relationship of our spirituality to the ordinary acts of eating, moving, and feeling, that is, to diet, exercise, and touch. These embodied issues are central to our spirituality and stewardship of God's gift of life. The redemption of our bodies and the health of our whole being require that we give attention to the ordinary and fundamental acts of embodiment, which are the medium and the ground for our spiritual adventures.

II. Soul Food and Spiritual Formation

As they journeyed toward the promised land, the Israelites were warned that two paths of life stood before them—the first path led to death and the second led to life. Without oversimplifying the nature of human and divine decision making, we too find ourselves facing two paths. Will we choose life and health or death and disease? Will we follow the divine bias toward health or turn toward habits and practices that injure both body and spirit? The counsel of God both then and now is to "choose life."

Diet figures prominently in the biblical story. The Israelites were called by God to be holy even as God is holy. Their holiness or "set apart-ness" was to be reflected in their ethical treatment of one another, in the observance of the sabbath, in hospitality to the stranger, and in their dietary habits. For reasons known to God alone, certain meats and fish were appropriate for consumption while others were taboo. What persons ate and their attitudes toward eating reflected their relationship to God.

Diet is also a matter of importance in the New Testament, most specifically in the writings of the apostle Paul. Paul's challenge to the strict adherence to Jewish dietary laws was grounded not in issues of health but in issues of ethics, equality, and theology. In Galatians, Paul asserts that Christian freedom may involve transcending a legalistic understanding of the Jewish dietary laws and the practice of circumcision. In Christ, there are neither unclean persons nor unclean foods. Our relationship to God is based on God's love for us, first of all, and not on any specific dietary prohibitions.

Nevertheless, Paul sees our eating habits as an issue of faith. To those Corinthians who saw issues of diet and lifestyle of little consequence, Paul asserts that our eating and drinking must be grounded in our participation in the "body of Christ" and our care for "the temple of God." "All things are lawful" to the Christian, "but not all things are helpful" (1 Corinthians 10:23).

What we eat, Paul counsels, may even have an impact on our neighbor. While we may "eat whatever is sold in the meat market without raising any question on the ground of conscience," even if this food is sacrificed to idols, we must take care that our eating and drinking is not a stumbling block to our "weaker" brother or sister (1 Corinthians 8:9–11).

Further, at the agape feasts of the Corinthian church, the rich came early, bringing the best food and wines, and then consumed their dinners before their more humble neighbors arrived. The agape feasts, Paul proclaims, are to mirror Christ's own eucharistic feast. While "food does not commend us to God" and "we are not worse off if we do not eat, and no better off if we eat" certain types of food, our eating must glorify God and bring us closer to our neighbor. The health of "the body of Christ" requires that our eating bring health to the souls of our neighbors and ourselves. Eating, as today's experts on world hunger suggest, has ethical consequences when it involves gluttony, on the one hand, and starvation, on the other. As Paul proclaims, "whether you eat or drink, or whatever you do, do all to the glory of God" (1 Corinthians 10:31).

While fasting has always been part of monastic spiritual formation and the practice of many devout laypersons, the nineteenth-century Seventh Day Adventist movement brought the issue of diet and abstinence once again to the forefront of Christian reflection. Although the the Adventist movement was ridiculed for its obsession with health and its expectation of the imminent Second Coming of Jesus, the dietary practices of the Seventh Day Adventists have been vindicated as contributors to health and well-being. Many of today's healthy diets, such as cardiologist Dean Ornish's "heart attack prevention diet" or the Pritikin diet, reflect the wisdom of Ellen B. White, the mother of the Adventist movement, and her disciples.

At the heart of Seventh Day Adventist thinking is the belief that what we eat has spiritual ramifications. Persons should live in accordance with the divine laws of health and embodiment. Ellen White asserted that the eating of meat, the use of tobacco, and the consumption of alcohol numb the mind and deaden the spirit. Many of us, sadly, can testify to this fact! The soul is most appropriately nourished by a diet consisting of grains, fruits, and vegetables—a far cry from the high fat and cholesterol diets of both the nineteenth century and today. The Adventists believed that we prepare ourselves for the Second Coming by presenting our bodies as "a living sacrifice" unto God and following God's laws of nutrition, rest, and exercise. The vegetarian orientation of the Seventh Day Adventists is reflected in longer lives and fewer cases of hypertension and heart disease, on average, than the fast food, meat-eating culture of most Americans. The God who resurrects the flesh on the last day is concerned with how we treat our flesh today!

In the spirit of the Adventist movement, Christians are discovering that diet is a matter of stewardship both of our own bodies and the bodies of others. Paul's gospel of Christian freedom did not, as some suggest, give Christians the license to eat whatever they want. Freedom in Christ leads to a responsible and loving life-style. We take care of the temple because it is part of God's creation and we affirm the bodies of others because they, too, are members of the body of Christ. We also recognize that irresponsible eating and drinking may lead to illnesses that burden our families, friends, and the social structure as well as tax the health resources available to our communities.

According to today's medical wisdom, what we eat and how we eat are matters of life and death. Dean Ornish and other physicians have noted that at least 50% of heart attacks and other forms of cardiovascular disease are related to life-style and eating habits. The traditional risk factors for heart disease and high blood pressure center around diet, lack of exercise, obesity, and smoking as well as age, gender, and genetics. We are a society plagued by cardiovascular disease: physicians estimate that sixty million Americans have some form of high blood pressure, hardening of the arteries, or heart disease.

Dean Ornish has been a pioneer in responding to heart disease in America. Ornish believes that the occurrence of cardiovascular disease may be an invitation to personal transformation. Through a transformed and healthy life-style, we can both reverse and prevent heart disease.[2] Ornish believes that the current medical focus on heart bypass operations simply *bypasses* the spiritual, emotional, and dietary issues that lead to cardiovascular disease. Prevention and recovery require a transformed mind and a commitment to life and health.

Ornish's program for healthy living involves a healthy diet, moderate exercise, quitting smoking, stress management, and spiritual formation. Ornish's diet follows closely the spirit of Adventist Ellen White. In contrast to the typical American diet, which is high in animal products, fat, cholesterol, salt, and sugar, Ornish advocates a diet emphasizing beans, legumes, fruits, grains, and vegetables, all of which are high in fiber and low in fat and cholesterol. If we are aware of what we eat, we can "eat more and weigh less" precisely because the foods we eat are low in fat and high in fiber. Further, as I will suggest later in this section, the Ornish and Adventist diets are also ecologically and morally sound, since the foods suggested are low on the food chain, require less processing, and, because of their vegetarian orientation, minimize the use of grain as animal feed. Many cookbooks today emphasize both a healthy diet and a healthy attitude toward the environment and the needs of persons in underdeveloped nations.[3]

Heart disease can be a catalyst for transformation insofar as it challenges us to rethink our priorities and choose new behaviors. An essential aspect of the Ornish program is "eating with mindfulness." While the term "mindfulness" has its origins in Buddhism, Christian leaders have also spoken of the importance of awareness and observation of our eating and of habitual behavior patterns in the process of spiritual formation. When we eat, we are challenged to eat slowly, tasting the food, and noting its impact on our bodies and minds. Ornish believes that many of our problems with food arise from the use of food to respond to emotional needs and our failure to listen to our bodies and their needs. The body has a wisdom that we disobey at our own peril. Andrew Weil, another physician concerned with health, asserts that what we eat and drink and our life-style can enhance or depress our body's natural healing processes.[4]

Most of us are virtually unaware of what we eat. How often have you eaten a meal while watching television, reading the paper, or planning the day ahead, and then, afterwards, asked yourself, "what did I just eat?" Clinical psychologist Elizabeth Wheeler notes that people often eat quickly and are surprised at how good food tastes, when they eat slowly and mindfully. When persons eat with awareness, "they're less likely to eat when they're not hungry, and less likely to eat beyond the point of fullness."[5]

Eating with mindfulness challenges today's Christian to choose between "fast food" and "soul food." This is not a matter of otherworldly salvation but a response to God's call to abundant life right now. In the spirit of Ornish and others, Christians can begin their personal transformation by exploring a spirituality of eating and serving. Such joyful and prayerful eating was at the heart of Jesus' table fellowship. Eating was as important as preaching for Jesus. He fed the five thousand, he ate with sinners and the wealthy, he transformed water into wine at Cana. Eating was a theological and ethical act that embodied God's love for the outcast and the sinful.

If we are to claim the spirit of Jesus' table fellowship, we must, first of all, surround our food with prayer. Too often, we cook, serve, and eat in a hurry. We pay little attention to our companions at the table. We barely notice the taste and are oblivious to the impact of certain foods on our well-being. We eat merely to "fill the void" or replenish an "empty gas tank." Our eating habits often negatively reflect our spiritual and emotional needs and disregard our nutritional and relational needs. Such compartmentalized and mechanistic eating habits lead to illness of both body and spirit.

Many liberal and mainstream Christians have abandoned mealtime prayer as archaic and repetitious. No doubt, some persons associate mealtime prayer with parental supervision, ritualistic repetition, or fundamentalist piety. In contrast, Jesus saw eating as a way of encountering God and trusting in God's bounty. Surrounding our meals with prayer can transform our food so that it becomes food for the spirit. It is an invitation to eat with an awareness that our diet is a spiritual issue. Today's Christians are called to follow the Native American image of eating in a holy and thankful way.

In my own cooking and food preparation, I seek to maintain a prayerful attitude. I follow the example of the kitchen mystic Brother Lawrence, who compared his time in the kitchen or shopping for supplies to his time spent at the eucharist.[6] I take time out to be thankful as I chop the vegetables, cut the fruit, or slice the chicken. I remember those for whom I am cooking and take a moment to pray for each one of them. If I become bothered or frustrated, I take a few breaths to center myself and ask that God be in my heart and mind as I cook and eat. While we do not always have regular mealtime blessings in my family, we try to spend the meal with one another in conversation and silence. We have learned the significance of doing one thing at a time and have, for the most part, broken the habit of "time sharing" our eating with the evening news and the sports page. Such times of family eating enable us to commune with one another in a more leisurely fashion and to discover what is important in each other's lives. As we surround our meals with blessing, our food becomes holy food, it becomes for us "the body and blood of Christ," and our spirits as well as our bodies are nurtured.

Eating is a form of celebrating the ordinariness of life. Surely this sort of celebration, which transforms the everyday into a celebration of God's presence, was at the heart of Jesus' own table fellowship. We can see this same celebration of the ordinary and the temporary in the Japanese tea ceremony, the celebration of the eucharistic elements of bread and wine, and the Navajo sand painting and hunting rituals. All these activities are transitory, but by our openness to the holy within these temporary events, we find personal balance and become part of the rhythms of nature and the divine.

Today, many Christians are reclaiming the ethical aspects of eating. In an era of widespread starvation, we must "live simply, so that others might simply live." Today, as we consume our processed foods and animal products (both of which contribute to cardiovascular illness), we must remember that other weight problem. As Ronald Sider states, "we are an affluent island in the midst of starving humanity."[7] Over one billion persons suffer from malnutrition. Over two hundred million children will suffer brain damage from lack of protein in their diet. The apostle Paul notes that one of the greatest, yet in our time forgotten, sins is gluttony. Today, as we heap our plates full at the bountiful buffet of fast foods and high cholesterol meals, we must turn our attention to those who beg for a morsel at the gates of the city all across the globe.

The prophet Amos once suggested that the wealthy and well fed will experience a "famine" of the word of God because of their injustice to the poor (Amos 8:11–12). Are we on the verge of such a famine? When we learn about the relationship between cattle raising and the destruction of the rainforest and the threat to the planetary ecosystem, we are convicted by the possibility that our current eating habits may jeopardize the survival of our children's children. Ronald Sider's suggestions for a "life-style of justice" are surprisingly similar to Ornish's counsels for a healthy life-style: substitute vegetable protein for animal protein, fast regularly, oppose the misuse of grain for beer and alcohol.[8]

Diet is both a personal and a social issue. An ethical and ecological diet is also a healthy diet. Since all of life is interdependent, what is good for the "body of Christ" as a totality is also good for each individual part! As we live more simply, we consciously share in the lives of others and experience our connectedness with the world beyond ourselves and our families. Isolationism in diet, life-style, and economics is unhealthy for ourselves and others. As we experience our connectedness with God and the body of Christ incarnate in our companions on the planet, we will begin to eat with a sense of holiness and care.

Many contemporary physicians suggest a completely vegetarian diet. I see nothing wrong with eating flesh sparingly and with mindfulness. But ask yourself how meat makes you feel. Which meat products add zest to your life and which depress your system? How do you feel about the killing of animals? We are not called to be dietary legalists, and there is no one norm to which we must conform. From time to time, I enjoy chicken and on occasion will order a steak. But, for reasons of ethics as well as health, these occasions are becoming more and more rare. We are called to be countercultural in our eating habits and to eat meaningfully and spiritually. Remember Paul's challenge to the Christians at Rome: "Be not conformed to the world, but be transformed by the renewing of your mind" (Romans 12:2). In addition to thanking God for the blessings of the hunt and the harvest, we are called to be grateful to the food itself as well as those who have prepared it for us.

Many Christians have found both a spiritual and a physical benefit in fasting. Fasting must be done, however, with care and discipline. When fasting becomes obsessive or injures our body, it violates the temple of God. Fasting is best employed when our motivation is to deepen our spiritual lives or live in solidarity with the poor and malnourished persons of our planet. Some persons contribute the money saved on fast days to local soup kitchens or hunger relief programs.

Fasting and other dietary practices should be done with grace and gentleness. For some, a fast supplemented by water will suffice; for others, juice is a necessity. Other persons, who require three regular meals to maintain their health or energy, can take time out before and after their meals to thank God for the gift of life and food and commit themselves to using their energy for the well-being of the neighborhood and the planet. Perhaps, the fast most appropriate for many of us who work long hours and lead busy lives is the abstinence from one meal, from time to time, or between meal or bedtime snacks. Such times, when devoted to God and our neighbor, are spiritual disciplines which focus the mind even as they relax the digestive system.

Diet is important in our spiritual and ethical formation. What we eat and how we eat can be a witness to our faith and a commitment to participating in God's healing work in our bodies and in the body of Christ. When we eat with mindfulness, ethical sensitivity, and gratitude, then every meal participates in Christ's own eucharistic feast.

III. Moving in the Spirit

While the Scriptures say much about diet, they are silent about exercise. Persons in nonindustrial societies seldom suffer from inactivity. It was normal for Jesus and his followers to carry heavy burdens and walk several miles a day. Tax collectors, carpenters, and priests did not have the benefit of automobiles, elevators, and buses. Only the royalty needed to look for ways to exercise either for fitness or pleasure. Nevertheless, the apostle Paul's words to the Athenians give us an image for a spirituality of exercise: "In God we live, move, and have our being" (Acts 17:28).

Today's Christians are challenged to find healthy ways to "move in the spirit." In a recent publication of the Shalem

Institute for Spiritual Formation in Washington D.C., spiritual guide Tilden Edwards states that "amazing things happen when our bodies join our minds in opening to God." In the past three decades, Christians have discovered the benefits of yoga postures for spiritual growth and physical well-being. Christians can take courses in body prayer and prayerful movement at spiritual institutes such as Shalem Institute. Through such practices, Christians can discover God's presence in the most ordinary of activities—sitting, walking, and standing.

Our attitude toward exercise is also a matter of choosing life or death. Inactivity is a major contributor to high blood pressure, heart attacks, and fatigue. Regular exercise, on the other hand, increases metabolism, promotes weight loss, reduces blood pressure, and decreases stress. Moderate exercise produces endorphins which promote optimism and feelings of emotional and spiritual well-being.

Pioneers in the spiritual care of persons with cancer, such as radiation oncologist O. Carl Simonton, prescribe regular exercise as a supplement to medical treatment, visualization, and counseling. Simonton has noted that persons unable to exercise due to their condition still reap physiological and spiritual benefits when they spend thirty minutes a day imaging themselves exercising.

In an era of "couch potatoes," Christians would do well to reflect on the words of the philosopher Plato:

There is no proportion or disproportion more productive of health and disease, and virtue and vice, than that between the soul and the body....There is one protection against disportion [of soul and body]—that we should not move the body without the soul, and the soul without the body, and thus they will be on their guard against each other and well balanced.[9]

Christians would also benefit from imitating Jesus, who spent much of his ministry outdoors walking from place to place, no doubt teaching, healing, and gathering information for his parables as he and his friends sojourned. We too might marvel at the lilies of the field and the birds of the air, if we spent more time in their company.

Although most people recognize the value of exercise as a means of promoting balance and good health, many people find exercise a meaningless burden and, despite their best intentions, fail to maintain any discipline of physical exercise. C.S. Lewis once noted that one of the marks of the Christian life is joy. In this spirit, we must discover joyful ways of caring for the temple of God. Exercise must be joined with spirituality and meaning, not fear and drudgery, if it is to promote wholeness of body and spirit. The irony of joyless exercise is found in a study that noted that although jogging may add a year to a person's life, preparing for jogging and jogging itself take up nearly a year of one's life over a thirty-year period.

Moving in the spirit is one of life's ordinary pleasures. Prayer and spiritual formation are not restricted to reading Scripture, sitting in meditation, or going to church. Today, persons are learning about "body prayer" (movements that accompany certain spoken or chanted prayers) as well as using their exercise time as a time of prayer and meditation. Herbert Benson suggests that the "relaxation response," a nonsectarian form of meditation I will describe more fully in the next chapter, can be joined with repetitive forms of exercise such as walking, swimming, or running. While one is walking, for example, one can focus on a particular repetitive word ("peace," "one," "God"). Benson notes that this approach to the "relaxation response" would be particularly interesting to pragmatic Americans, insofar as it combines stress reduction, exercise, and spiritual growth![10]

Moving in the spirit, as Tilden Edwards suggests, begins

with an awareness of our bodies. One non-aerobic form of moving meditation encouraged by Edwards is walking meditation. In walking meditation, one moves quietly and gently with an awareness of each movement and the wondrous intricacy of our being.

When we move in the spirit, we discover that exercise can be both meaningful and joyful. Each person must discover the discipline proper to one's particular physical condition and personal characteristics. My own choice involves walking and jogging. Each morning, after my morning meditation, I sojourn on a four-mile, one-hour walk, along the creek near my home in Bethesda, Maryland. I use the time of walking as a continuation of my morning meditation.

Some mornings, I take a moment to read the lectionary readings for the Sunday services. As I walk, I roll the images and ideas in my mind. I've discovered that insights, questions, and responses come effortlessly as I quietly walk in my neighborhood. Other mornings, I choose to participate in a fast-walking meditation. As I move along at four miles an hour, I simply let my prayer word guide me. When my mind wanders, as it often does, I bring it gently back. Still other days, I image God's healing light entering and surrounding my body with each breath. I experience the light of God bringing me wisdom, intelligence, health, truthfulness, creativity, and forgiveness as I focus on the various "energy centers" of the body. Before an important talk or lecture, I often walk around the block imaging the room, praying for the participants, and asking for God's guidance. By the time I arrive, I usually feel calm and centered in God's presence.

Walking can also be an invitation to appreciation. As I walk, I often merely gaze upon the trees, listen to the stream, or hear the cars. As I pass a fellow walker, I say a brief prayer that God blesses them. Dr. Robert Perry, pastor of North Chevy Chase Christian Church (Disciples of Christ) in Chevy Chase,

Maryland, tells of a woman in his church who spends her daily walk simply thanking God for each blessing she has received. Although her life has been far from easy, she claims never to have run out of things for which to be thankful. I have joined thanksgiving and intercession in my own walking and have found myself blessed as I bless others. In the spirit of Jesus' walking fellowship, we can affirm with the Navajo, "with beauty all around me, I walk."

Walking also joins us with other persons. Virtually every evening, I walk a few miles with my wife or teenage son Matt. I learned this discipline from walks with my father during my college days. In the gentleness of our walks, as our beagle Fred tags along, we often have the leisure to discuss dreams and challenges, or just to share the silence. In a time in which our lives are often dominated by work, noise, and busyness, walking provides an opportunity for a family to communicate with one another. Time slows down and we experience a glimpse of eternity in the world of passing time.

In recent years, Christians have sought to integrate spirituality with aerobic exercise. A former parishioner at Georgetown University now teaches aerobics in a program called "Body and Soul." This program combines dynamic exercise with prayer, fellowship, and Christian music. Each session has a particular theme such as praise, Christian unity, victory in Christ, and outreach, which serves to affirm and encourage persons on their spiritual journey. Such meaningful exercise provides both spiritual and physical benefits, in a supportive and nonjudgmental environment. Today, the church is called to be a place of healing and recreation, where persons can integrate faith and action in the most literal way possible in the integration of exercise, fellowship, and inspiration.

Moving in the spirit is ultimately a way to experience God's grace in the world of the flesh. We care for our bodies in response to God's gift of embodiment. As we bring God into our eating, touching, working, playing, and exercise, we will experience an integrated and balanced life. Our own lives will be attuned to God's life as we discover, moment by moment, what it means to "pray without ceasing."

IV. In Touch With God

Today, a great deal of controversy surrounds the use of touch in healing and pastoral relationships. While touch is essential to human well-being, touch can also manipulate, dehumanize, and abuse. Many persons today not only suffer the effects of abusive touch, they also suffer from touch deprivation. Studies have found that infants who are not touched or seldom touched have higher incidences of illness and death than those who are regularly caressed and fondled. Such studies have led to creative ways of responding to infants in neonatal intensive care units. As Julie Denison suggests in an article in *Christian Century,* what is needed today is "not less, but a different kind of touch."[11] In that spirit, all of my reflections on the relationship of touch and healing are grounded in the awareness that touch is healing only when it is safe, creative, freely received, and nonmanipulative. Christians must challenge the destructive use of touch in pastoral relationships, sexual abuse, pornography, and physical abuse, even as we explore new and healthy patterns of touch and physical expression. Destructive touch objectifies and stereotypes, while creative, healing touch recognizes holiness, unity, and uniqueness.

In describing the importance of touch, Ashley Montagu noted that "next to the brain, the skin is the most important of our organ systems."[12] John Naisbitt, the author of *Megatrends,* claims that "the more technology is around us, the more the need for healing touch."[13] The key word is "healing" touch. Touch is healing when it enables us to experience wholeness and connectedness with God at a physical, spiritual, and emotional level. As the healing ministry of Jesus makes clear, healing touch heightens our awareness of God's presence in our bodies and activates the body's own natural tendencies toward healing. Healing touch feeds both the body and the spirit.

The healer Jesus, as we will see in chapter five, used a variety of methods to bring people to emotional, physical, and spiritual wholeness. Central to Jesus' healing was the embodiment of love through healing touch. New life is imparted and old wounds healed when Jesus touches Jairus' deceased daughter, a man born born blind, Peter's mother-in-law suffering from a fever, and Malchus' severed ear. Jesus' own skin was a medium of healing. When the woman suffering from a chronic hemorrhage touches him, Jesus experiences great power going forth from himself into the faithful woman.

Our skin both expresses and reveals our emotional life each time we blush. Massage therapists, bioenergetic practitioners, and other touch therapists have even found that touch elicits memories and brings healing to old emotional wounds. Studies have found that dogs exhibit positive physiological responses when they are petted. Persons who own dogs and cats tend to live longer and healthier lives, not only because of the feelings of warmth toward their animals but also because of the regular stroking of the four-footed friends. When we are connected emotionally and physically with another being, human or nonhuman, we experience greater connection with the love at the root of all being.

Today's Christians need to revive the ministry of healing touch both informally and through body-affirming disciplines.

Massage is, perhaps, the most readily available form of healing touch. Whether through gently rubbing one's own or another's sore neck or using more sophisticated forms of acupressure on the body's energy points, massage reduces stress, brings relaxation to the muscles, stimulates blood circulation, strengthens the immune system, and enhances complexion. Such simple forms of self-massage or acupressure can be practiced by virtually anyone, regardless of physical condition. Persons who are out of touch with their bodies may discover the pleasures of embodiment through massage.

Embraces and hugs also enhance well-being. When hugs are given in an affirming and healing manner they reconnect us with one another and ground us in our relationships. Sadly, many persons living alone go through days and weeks without being touched. Such touch deprivation, especially among the widowed elderly and single persons, depresses the immune system and may lead, in some persons, to inappropriate touching of others. The sign of peace in church should be a time of holy touch and affirmation of one another as God's children.

Today, at many hospitals, nurses and other caregivers are learning about "therapeutic touch." Introduced by Dolores Krieger, a professor of nursing at New York University, therapeutic touch has been shown to relieve pain, reduce swelling, enable bones to heal more quickly, and encourage sleep. In contrast to massage, therapeutic touch focuses on the energy field approximately six inches beyond the skin. It is believed that our embodiment goes beyond our skin and radiates into the field beyond our bodies. Our energy fields both reflect and nourish our physical and spiritual well-being. Therapeutic touch is an easily learned five-step process.

1. Centering, or opening to God and the forces of wholeness through prayer and meditation.

2. Assessment of a person's energy field in order to discern places of imbalance or depletion.

3. Clearing the blockages through downward sweeping

motions of the hands, which literally brush away imbalances.

4. Filling the holes, or bringing new energy to depleted areas.

5. Balancing the energy field, by sweeping the excess energy away from the body.

In connecting us to the divine energy of life, therapeutic touch brings renewed health, new efficiency, and greater creativity to those who give and receive treatments.[14] While Scripture says nothing about auras or energy fields, some scholars have likened the the power of *pneuma* (breath or spirit) to the Chinese understanding of *chi* or energy, which is at the heart of acupuncture.

In my own journey toward embodied spirituality, the practice of "reiki" has been the central discipline. Reiki (based on the root word *ki* or *chi*) means simply "universal or divine energy." Divine energy is all around us, the visible and invisible expression of the God in whom we "live, move, and have our being." The practice of reiki is one means of gently and unobtrusively channeling or sharing the healing energy of God and, in so doing, enhancing the healing movements in ourselves and others.

While the discovery of reiki is shrouded in mystery, one version sees its origins in the spiritual journey of a Christian minister and academic, Dr. Mikao Usui. In the late nineteenth century, Usui served as minister and principal at a Christian school in Kyoto, Japan. Following one of his sermons, his pupils challenged him with a life-changing question. They asked him if Jesus' healings really occurred. When Usui responded positively, they challenged him to produce a healing. His inability to practice what he preached led Usui on a spiritual journey which took him to a divinity school in the United States, a Buddhist monastery, the study of Indian healing texts, and a mystical experience that gave him the power and the courage to become a healer. In his own healing journey, Usui discovered a healing methodology that had been abandoned by ascetic Buddhism and scorned by rationalistic Christianity.

Although reiki's discovery was in Japan, it has now made its way across the planet and is a bridge between Christianity, Buddhism, and the more embodied healing technologies of the new age movement. According to the philosophy of reiki, we exist in a sea of divine, healing energy. We thirst for healing only because we do not know how to contact the waters of healing that surround us. The practice of reiki, its training and initiation, though very modest, opens us up in unexpected ways to resources of healing and stress release. Reiki, in its most basic form, is almost entirely "hands on." By gently touching various parts of the body, the reiki practitioner mediates or channels energy that both balances and heals. The energy clearly does not come from the practitioner. He or she is only the medium for its movement.

As gentle and undramatic as reiki is, it produces some surprising effects. A former reiki student of mine used reiki to treat a broken hip. Her physician was amazed at her rapid recovery. She had healed more quickly than any patient he had ever treated. Another practitioner I know experienced virtually no side effects following abdominal surgery, which she attributed to her own self-reiki and the "hands on" reiki of a friend who accompanied her to the hospital. Another friend uses reiki to ease the pain of persons in the final stages of AIDS. I have often given reiki treatments to persons undergoing psychological and spiritual stress or experiencing the pain of recently surfaced memories. Such encounters have brought a sense of calm and peace as well as hope for future healing.

Reiki is a way of life. The practice of reiki has become central to my own spiritual journey. As a reiki master/teacher and practitioner for ten years, I begin each day with my own self-healing. After my morning time of silence, I give myself a ten-minute treatment, beginning with my forehead and working my way down to my prostate. During the day, I often give a quick treatment to my wife, child, or a friend. The use of reiki has awakened me to the experience of all touch as a means of grace and healing. At least once or twice each day, I will give a "distant" reiki treatment to someone undergoing surgery or personal anguish. Like intercessory prayer, reiki is not bound by time or place. Its healing energy radiates across the universe.

When I give a reiki treatment, I image God's healing light flowing through me into the body of the other. Today, reiki is one of the most "holistic" of the alternative or complementary healing approaches. While it is expressed in touch, it is grounded in spiritual centeredness. In its embodiedness, reiki is a witness to the mind-spirit-body-emotional unity that brings healing to every level of our being and to the grace of God's healing energy in action.

V. Caring for the Temple

In contrast to the body denial of Gnostic spiritualities, both ancient and modern, Christian faith proclaims that the body is made by love and for love. In loving our bodies, we are loving the Creator whose love radiates through us. In nurturing the bodies of others, we are expressing God's love—we are, as the saying goes, "God's hands and God's feet." We are expressing God's desires for the universe in the microcosm of our own lives and encounters.

This chapter is an invitation for you to explore and experience the wonder of embodiment. My focus on certain techniques and omission of others is not meant to discount other diets, forms of exercise, or healing modalities. I believe that wherever healing occurs, God is present and Christ is alive, even if God's name is explicitly not invoked. All paths of healing, be they hands on, technological, Christian, or Asian, have their origins in the unconditional and unfettered love of God. As Christians, we are free to use prayer and prozac, reiki and radiation, massage and multivitamins.

Further, although I have not discussed sexuality in this chapter, I am convinced that life-supporting sexual intimacy is also a means by which we experience God's grace mediated through the embodiment of our partner and ourselves. Sexuality is essential to our well-being, whether our intimacy involves sexual intercourse in the context of a committed relationship or life-affirming celibacy. In an era of AIDS, sexual abuse, professional misconduct, and pornography, the church is challenged to explore the relationship of sexuality to spiritual formation.

As we learn more about the mind-body connection, we will, as the early Christians, find ourselves in world of "signs and wonders." As W.H. Auden proclaims in his Christmas Oratorio, *For the Time Being*:

He is the Way.
Follow Him through the land of Unlikeness;
You will see rare beasts, and have unique adventures.

He is the truth.
Seek Him in the kingdom of Anxiety;
You will come to a great city that has expected your return for years.

He is the Life.
Love him in the World of the Flesh; And at your marriage all its occasions shall dance for joy.[15]

QUESTIONS FOR REFLECTION AND DISCUSSION

1) How do you understand the spiritual and ethical dimensions of eating?

2) How would you describe your own eating patterns? Are you often able to eat mindfully?

3) How do you relate faith and exercise?

4) How have you experienced touch as a means of healing and grace?

5) Do you think that it is possible to integrate Christian forms of healing, such as laying on of hands, with Asian techniques such as acupuncture?

6) What is the theological meaning of loving God in "the world of the flesh?"

CHAPTER THREE

STRESSED, BUT NOT DISTRESSED

I. Stress and the Spirit

This morning, as usual, I began my day with a meditative stroll along Little Falls Creek near my home in Bethesda, Maryland. My heart was still and my spirit at peace as I breathed in God's presence and began my time of personal reflection and walking meditation. But my peace was quickly interrupted, not by the sounds of the waking city, but by the babble of my own mind. I began to reflect on all I had to do that day and the many tasks that I needed to accomplish before the new semester began. As I rehearsed the list, my body reflected my inner turmoil—my heart beat faster and my mind reeled at the thought the near impossible deadlines I had imposed upon myself.

Every day, we discover how easy it is to become "stressed out" and how our thoughts and emotions have an immediate impact on our bodily and spiritual well-being. Often, as I eat my lunch on the steps of Healy Hall at Georgetown University, I am struck by the grim determination of the students and staff who pass my noontime oasis. There is little joy and much obvious anxiety. When I ask a student how she is doing, rather than telling me how she feels, typically she recites a long list of projects and things to do and concludes with "I just don't know how I'm going to get all this done." I was astounded a number of years ago when my own son, then only in the fourth grade, complained of being stressed out. In our day, stress and other forms of emotional fatigue are epidemic and, in some circles, the degree of one's stress is considered a sign of diligence and commitment! A peaceful and centered spirit is somehow seen to be counterproductive or un-American.

In the previous chapter, I focused on the theology of embodiment. I suggested that how we treat our bodies is a matter of faith and unfaith. The same dynamic applies to our spiritual and emotional lives. Proverbs proclaims that "as a person thinks, therefore he or she is." Despite the philosophical dualism of Descartes and the compartmentalization characteristic of many forms of medicine, education, and religion today, physicians and laypersons alike are discovering that there is no ultimate split between mind and body. Every aspect of our lives exists in dynamic interrelatedness with all the others. Scientists as well as theologians are also discovering that there is no sharp dividing line between thoughts, emotions, and physical experiences. For good or for ill, the body is a mirror of our thoughts and emotions. A fantasy can soothe us or drive us into panic. An image can literally make us sick. Neuroimmunologists have discovered that peptides, neurotransmitters whose purpose is to transfer information and emotion, are found in the intestinal lining as well as in the brain. So, our thoughts are embodied and our bodies are inspired! As physician Bernie Siegel claims, "body and mind are different expressions of the same information."[1]

Long before quantum physics or the holistic medicine

movement, Jesus and his followers realized that faith and unfaith can be a matter of life and death. Our feelings about ourselves, others, and God can cure or kill. Today, we are challenged to nurture a faith that makes us whole in an increasingly complicated and fragmented world.

Stress, or the response to any challenge in life, has become a significant problem for modern persons. Although death is, as Hans Selye states, the only insurance against stress, many persons find themselves not only stressed, but distressed and "burned out" as they succumb to the diseases of modern civilization. Some physicians have concluded that 75-90% of all illness is stress-related and, of course, stress-related illness only produces further stress. Stress has been found to contribute to ailments as diverse as ulcers, acne, asthma, hypertension, heart attacks, arthritis, and cancer. In this chapter, I am broadening the clinical definition of stress to include the spiritual and emotional responses to agitating thoughts, emotions, or memories that challenge our current self-image or emotional, spiritual, and physical lives. Stress is one of the many ways our minds and emotions place heavy burdens on our physical well-being. Stress, accordingly, may be brought about by good news (a new job or a wanted pregnancy); it may also arise from bad news (the memory of physical or sexual abuse or the loss of a job). Stress, and its accompanying wear and tear on the body, may be brought about by hopelessness and passivity as well as anxiety and impatience.

One of the most significant causes of stress is our perception of time. In the early 1960s I recall watching a program describing the wonders of life in the 1990s. The commentator reflected on how persons in the 1990s would cope with all the extra leisure time that would result from labor-saving devices. Virtually everyone, the show suggested, would work fewer hours and would have more time for family life, travel, and personal growth. As I look at life in the 1990s, it is obvious how naive and idealistic such prognostications were. Today, persons work longer hours and commute greater distances. Computers, fax machines, E-mail—all of which were meant to simplify our lives—have made our lives more complicated and threaten to drown us in a sea of apparently essential information. Labor-saving devices become stress-producers when their complexity overwhelms us or when, for reasons known only to the machines themselves, they malfunction. (This week, I experienced the stress of the information highway firsthand, when my two new computers, one at the office and the other at home, both deleted my revisions of the first chapter of this book! I know that I am not the only victim of computer-induced stress and hypertension!) Most couples struggle to integrate full-time jobs with parenting and are constantly on the run from the office to school to the grocery store to sports practice. There is little time for unplanned conversations with children or neighbors. Even the search for community and spirituality has become stressful for those persons who agonize about their need to find some quiet time for prayer and meditation or extra time for exercise or going to church.

Today, many persons suffer from "hurry sickness." Like the white rabbit of *Alice's Adventures in Wonderland,* we are "late, late, for a very important date." Even if we're not entirely sure where we're going or why we wish to go there, we are pushed along by the momentum of our thoughts, projects, and expectations.

"Hurry" or "time sickness" finds its origins in the external or internal pressures to "beat the clock" and make "the deadline." Hurry sickness, a term used by physician Larry Dossey, is a factor in hypertension and contributes to high cholesterol, as studies of accountants in the weeks before April 15 suggest. It also leaves us with a vague spiritual and physical uneasiness, often expressed in migraines, back and neck aches, shortness of breath and heaviness in the chest, indigestion, and the inability to relax and enjoy life after work or on holidays.

Hurry sickness, like all forms of stress, is a spiritual issue, grounded in how we view the nature of time. Is time the mere passage of one moment to another or is time a reflection of meaning and purpose? Is our perspective on time seen in light of milliseconds and eight-hour days or the work of a whole lifetime or God's own timetable? As medical studies indicate, how we view time may also be a matter of life and death! Further, in another context, time may be a source of disease insofar as memories of the past and past conditioning may come to dominate the present moment's possibilities for growth and adventure.

As we will see, many of the stresses of life are grounded in the perception of scarcity. Persons today often feel they do not have enough time, energy, intelligence, and support to prosper and flourish in their daily lives. Isolated and disconnected from the spiritual wellsprings of life, they feel bereft of resources to face the challenges of the day or the times. Yet, as I will suggest, the spiritual vision of life proclaims an alternative understanding of reality—one grounded in the perception of abundance and the recognition that each person is connected to a higher creativity and infinite wisdom and care that supports and nurtures them at all times. This infinite wellspring, the power of God, is available to all persons all the time, but empowers us most fully when we "ask, seek, and knock" for its help and guidance. This alternative vision is at the heart of Jesus' admonition to his stressed-out followers both then and now:

> Therefore, I tell you, do not be anxious about your life, what you shall eat and what you shall drink, nor about your body, what you shall put on....Look at the birds of the air, they neither sow nor reap nor gather into barns,

and yet your heavenly Father feeds them....Consider the lilies of the field, how they grow, they neither toil nor spin; yet, I tell you, even Solomon in all his glory was not arrayed like one of these. But, if God so clothes the grass of the field, which today is alive and tomorrow is thrown into the oven, will God not much more clothe you, O persons of little faith?....But, seek first God's kingdom and God's righteousness and all these shall be yours as well. (Matthew 6:25–26,28–30,33)

One of the greatest spiritual challenges for persons today is to trust God's care for the totality of their lives. Apart from such trust our lives become fragmented and anxious and our spiritual dis-ease soon becomes manifest in physical breakdown. We must discover creative ways to be stressed without becoming distressed!

II. The Dangers of Distress

Cancer and heart disease are the two greatest killers of our time. Medical educators have long identified certain life-styles that increase one's likelihood of cancer and heart disease: diet, smoking, lack of exercise, environmental factors, obesity, and genetic tendencies. In recent years, other researchers have reflected on the nonquantifiable, emotional, and spiritual aspects of cancer and heart disease. Certain persons who habitually exhibit all the risk behaviors flourish, while others with the same risk factors succumb. Can such differences be solely a matter of chance or good luck, or is there a spiritual component to the susceptibility and prevention of cancer, heart disease, and other ailments?

As they reflect on the spiritual and emotional components of health and illness, certain alternative healers contend that health and illness are almost entirely a matter of conscious or unconscious choice. New age healers such as Louise Hay claim that persons "create their own realities" and that each person is "100% responsible for their health and illness."[2] In the same spirit, certain Christian healers suggest that the faithful can "name and claim it." Good health is a sign of faithfulness, while disease and inability to get well have their ultimate basis in lack of faith. Such images of personal omnipotence are both theologically wrong and emotionally dangerous. In "blaming the victim," they inspire feelings of guilt and hopelessness which only further depress the immune system. Further, by suggesting that our faith alone is responsible for health and illness, they neglect the ecological and relational nature of health as well as God's role in healing the sick. Health becomes a matter of what the Protestant Reformers called "works righteousness." Nevertheless, the impact of our emotional and spiritual lives cannot be underestimated both in the prevention and the healing of disease. Lawrence LeShan, a psychologist who pioneered the studies in spirituality and cancer, suggests that, even if emotional factors play only a 5% role in health, illness, and recovery, "we know that 5% can make a difference—in a hard fought election."[3]

According to many students of psychosomatic or whole-person medicine, no disease reflects "hurry sickness" more than heart disease. As a result of his study of persons who sought his care following heart attacks, Dr. Meyer Friedman originated the concept of the "Type A" personality. The majority of Friedman's patients were highly competitive, impatient, and hardworking. Although initially heart disease was identified with "workaholic" behaviors, later studies modified this conclusion. The stress of life, which may lead to heart disease, is not merely a result of long hours and commitment to one's job, it is related to how one perceives one's work and the world.[4]

Type A personalities tend to perceive the world as basically hostile and indifferent. In a graceless world, the only appropriate philosophy of life is that of football coach Vince Lombardi, "winning is the *only* thing!" It is absolutely essential to be *in control* in an out-of-control and chaotic world. Ironically, the more one seeks to be in control, the more one's emotional life is controlled by external events. When I am late for a meeting, every chance encounter is a nuisance, every slow driver is an enemy, and every red light is witness to the malevolence of the universe. My hand, like a revolver, is poised near the horn at every intersection! My body reflects this anxiety through shallow breathing and stomach acid. In contrast, when I perceive the world as abundant in time and energy, I see every encounter as a blessing and an invitation to adventure and every red light as an opportunity to enjoy the scenery and take time for brief prayers and affirmations. Mirroring my state of mind and spirit, my body feels rested even in a rush hour traffic jam.

Ultimately, the Type A personality becomes a spiritual issue. Even if there is a God, the world is perceived to be untrustworthy and each person is on his or her own. Isolated from one another in a world in which my neighbor's gain is my loss, the Type A person believes his or her best hope for survival and well-being is to take care of her or himself first and foremost. Like a branch severed from the nourishment of the vine, such an individual perceives little or no likelihood of divine or interpersonal support in the realization of personal hopes and dreams.

Connectedness with life is absolutely essential for emotional, spiritual, and physical well-being. Without connectedness to our mothers, we could not survive. Apart from the care that leads to what psychiatrist Erik Erikson calls "basic trust," the universe seems at best indifferent and at worst hostile. Type A philosophy is in radical contrast to the relational image of life, portrayed in Paul's image of the "body of Christ" where everyone can count on a supportive environment in which "if one member suffers, all suffer together; if one member rejoices, all rejoice together" (1 Corinthians 12:26).

In his groundbreaking work on the relationship between emotions and heart disease, James Lynch suggests that our relationships are a matter of life and death.[5] In virtually every disease category, single, widowed, and divorced persons have higher mortality rates than those who are married. Accordingly, social isolation and lack of companionship, whether it be due to death, divorce, work style, or philosophy of life, may be a significant factor in premature death. Lynch notes that studies of mortality rates indicate that religious involvement is a factor in health and longevity. Men who frequently attend church have a 60% lower mortality rate than those who do not; women who are involved in church life have a 50% lower mortality rate. I would suggest that whether the difference in mortality rate is due to belonging to a community or one's relationship to God, the issue is ultimately one of connection to a trustworthy and supportive reality. The churchgoing person experiences at a conscious (as well as unconscious) level a life-supporting sense of connection not only with others (persons in worship, Bible studies, choir, and fellowship groups), but also a greater connection with God and the universe.

Albert Einstein once suggested that the most important question a person can ask is, "is the universe friendly or not?" To believe in God as one's intimate companion is ultimately to see the universe and the framework of our personal lives as supportive, friendly, and trustworthy. It is also to claim that one's life is not defined by one moment, one day, or one lifetime, but by eternity. Those who see the world as chaotic and meaningless are like those branches, in Jesus' sermon, that are disconnected from the vine (John 15:6). Connectedness to God and the other branches is a matter of life and death spiritually and physically, "for apart from me, you can do nothing" (John

15:5). In contrast, those who abide in Christ and open themselves to the resources of a supportive universe "bear much fruit" (John 15:8). The challenge for persons today is to find appropriate pathways and disciplines in order to nurture connectedness with God and their neighbors.

Feelings of disconnectedness also contribute to the stresses that may bring about the incidence of cancer. According to many cancer researchers, cancer is a prime example of a dysfunctional mind-body relationship. Carl Simonton, a radiation oncologist, suggests that "we all participate in our health through our beliefs, feelings, and attitudes toward life, as well as more direct ways such as exercise and diet."[6] Simonton states that illness is "not purely a physical problem but a problem of the whole person...emotional and mental states play a significant role in the susceptibility of disease, including cancer, and the recovery from all disease."[7]

Researchers describe a constellation of personality traits that may be related to the incidence of cancer. Lawrence LeShan notes that in many of the patients he has treated prior to the diagnosis of cancer, there has been "a loss of hope in ever achieving a way of life that would give real and deep satisfaction, that would provide a solid *raison d'être*, a kind of meaning that makes us glad to get out of bed in the morning and glad to go back to bed at night—the kind of life that makes us look forward to each day and to the future."[8] LeShan has found a loss of hope in 70-80% of the hundreds of persons with cancer he has treated. He elaborates that "persons with cancer, I believe, died from a negative state of stress, so to speak. They die when they are overcome by a state of futility and hopelessness."[9]

When one has no hope for transformation and feels disconnected from any significant spiritual or emotional support, the immune system breaks down and can no longer identify and destroy the cancer cells that inhabit the body. Whereas the

Type A personality is characterized by competitiveness and the perception of a hostile world, the cancer-prone personality is characterized by lack of meaning, inability to express feelings, emotional dissociation, hopelessness about change, and lack of faith in the ability of relationships to be supportive and healing.[10] Simonton and others have gone so far as to note certain specific chronological and childhood precursors to the incidence of cancer: 1) childhood experiences that lead to an inability to trust and seek support from other persons, 2) a major personal stress (divorce, loss of employment), 3) inability to respond creatively to the crisis given one's habitual coping skills, 4) feelings of being trapped and unable to change, 5) avoidance of the problem.[11]

The spiritual dimension of cancer reflects feelings of alienation, disconnectedness, and rigidity. In her or his hopelessness, the cancer-prone person perceives the universe to be both unconcerned and unsupportive. Neither God nor other persons can provide the resources one needs not only to live but to live abundantly and zestfully.

Chronic and deep-seated spiritual and emotional disconnectedness suppresses the ability of the immune system both to identify and to eliminate cancer cells. Like a branch disconnected from the vitality of the vine, the body and spirit wither and cancer gains a foothold. Even with the best of medical care, the hope for survival ultimately lies in the possibility of spiritual transformation—the emergence of a "new creation," a new orientation on life that enables one to begin to trust God, other persons, and one's ability to change.

In this section, I have explored the spiritual dimensions of heart disease and cancer. These same dimensions apply to many other ailments of body and spirit. Feelings of disconnectedness play an important role in both the conscious and unconscious behaviors and attitudes that lead to the breakdown of the cardiovascular and immune systems. In my emphasis on these factors, I do not intend to blame the victim, since illness results from many factors, rather than merely our own bodily constitution, behaviors, or thoughts. The final word is not hopelessness or guilt, but the possibility of transformation, new life, and grace. However, it is clear that if there is no boundary between body, mind, spirit, and environment, our attitudes and spiritual commitments can be decisive in health and illness. When we discover the importance of spirituality in health and illness, we can actively orient our lives toward spiritual well-being. We can prevent illness as well as "get well again." Still, our commitment to and participation in spiritual disciplines is as important to overall well-being and preventative care as diet and exercise.

III. Not Conformed, But Transformed

Faith is ultimately countercultural in nature. The apostle Paul counseled his parishioners, "be not conformed to the world, but be transformed by the renewing of your mind." In his New Testament translation, J.B. Phillips suggest an alternative, "do not let the world squeeze you into its mold." As we reflect on the issue of holistic health and healing, the term "world" does not indicate the physical universe created by God, but relates to all those attitudes, behavior patterns, family myths and practices, and social mores that prevent us from becoming fully alive and fully open to God's healing presence in our lives. The world we must transform is the world of rigid behavior patterns, unhealed memories, inauthentic and destructive values, and unhealthy life-styles. Choosing the path of spiritual and physical well-being requires constant transformation and the willingness to follow the path of life and healing rather than the path of social convention and dysfunctional life-style.

Today, Christians must be globally prophetic. We must seek alternatives to the way of death in economics by immersing ourselves in journals such as *Salt, Sojourners,* and *The Other Side,* by "thinking globally and acting locally" for peace and justice, and by transforming our individual and corporate spiritual lives. As the Church of the Savior in Washington D.C. has long advised, we must "journey inward" and "journey outward" if our world is to be healed.

The key element in this transformation is the "renewing of the mind," the commitment to see the world and our lives from a new and broader perspective. The healing of relationships, memories, habits, that breaks the cycle of stress results from a commitment to holistic spiritual practices and a faith in the resourcefulness of a God "who makes a way when there is no way." On our own and disconnected from the vitality of the "vine," we have few resources for the radical changes that are necessary. Spiritual transformation requires a faith in our personal resources for change grounded in our connectedness to God and other persons of faith. As Paul proclaims, "I can do all things," not on my own or in isolation from others, but "through Christ who strengthens me."

Recently, a friend of mine participated in a firewalking retreat. At first, she was both fearful and incredulous. How can a person walk across coals heated to nearly 1200 degrees Fahrenheit? To the pessimist and the realist, such an act is an impossibility. But, there is a deeper reality than what meets the eyes. Persons walk across the coals as a result of the spiritual discipline that leads to a transformed mind. In preparation for the firewalk, persons face their fears, open to the greater spiritual resources in themselves, and ground themselves in the experience of the present moment. The only way to walk on the coals is to walk in power and trust one step at a time. Each of us must make our own firewalk as we seek health and healing. For us, the fire we face may not be the result of blistering coals, it may be a lack of self-esteem, an unhealed memory, the diagnosis of a serious illness, or personal depression. We

know that the cost of stagnation, hopelessness, and disconnectedness may be illness and death, both spiritual and physical. Choosing life means a commitment to transformation.
But this commitment comes only when we trust God, even in
our unbelief, and when, with all our doubts, we affirm with
the apostle Paul, "Christ in me, the hope of glorious things to
come" as we journey through the crisis one step at a time.

In the following paragraphs, we will explore four disciplines of holistic spiritual transformation. Although these disciplines do not necessarily require physical movement, they
are deeply embodied and incarnational in nature. While many
spiritual disciplines lead to wholeness of body, mind, and spirit, the disciplines of sabbath time, meditation for stress reduction and spiritual growth, visualization, and affirmation
ground us deeply in the interplay of body and spirit, hope and
realism. They enable us not only to avoid distress but also to
transform stress into strength.

1. *The Sanctuary of Time.* Our attitude toward time is a major
cause of stress in modern life. While the passage of time is an
essential aspect of reality, modern persons often see the natural flow of time as a threat to their well-being. But the passage
of time is the ground of growth, creativity, novelty, and transformation. From the spiritual perspective, time is spacious and
abundant. There is always enough time for birth, growth, and
fruition.

The modern world, in contrast to the world of spiritual
abundance, has defined time as ultimately linear, discrete, and
one-dimensional. From this vantage point, time becomes a
commodity that is always running down. Confronted by
deadlines and constantly consulting their timepieces, modern
persons never have enough time. In focusing on the discrete
and linear nature of time, persons become disconnected from
the past and anxious about the future. Such a vision of time

leads to hurry sickness and the inability to live fully in the present moment. Death and its "sting" become the primary fear as well as motivation for those who live solely by clock time. Aging becomes an enemy to be defeated and denied, a visible manifestation of scarcity rather than a revelation of growing wisdom.

There is, however, an antidote to hurry sickness. This antidote is found in our awakening to *kairos* or sabbath time. *Kairos* time, in contrast to *chronos* or clock time, is the "full," "ripe," and "abundant" time of God. The Hebrews saw *kairos* time in terms of the sabbath. In response to God's creative and liberating work in the cosmos and human history, the Hebrew people were called to:

> Remember the sabbath day, to keep it holy. Six days you shall labor, and do all your work. But, the seventh day is a sabbath to the Lord your God; in it you shall not do any work, you, or your son, or your daughter, your man-servant or your maidservant, or your cattle or the sojourner who is in your gates; for in six days the Lord made heaven and earth, the sea and all that is in them, and rested the seventh day; therefore the Lord blessed the sabbath day and hallowed it (Exodus 20:8–11).

The sabbath of creation reflects God's own personal sabbath. At the end of God's work, God rested and, as some translations suggest, was refreshed (Genesis 2:2). While the true meaning of the sabbath has often been lost through legalistic attitudes toward rest and work, the sabbath nevertheless points to the importance of rest and worship in the spiritual life. Abraham Heschel speaks of the sabbath as a "sanctuary of time."[12] At times of rest, we experience the "eternal in time" and have the "opportunity to mend our tattered lives."[13] In days and moments of quiet, we are enabled to reconnect with

God. Such moments and days not only recharge our spiritual lives, they also replenish our immune and cardiovascular systems. In letting go of control, our whole being rests and re-creates itself. Even Jesus, who often critiqued legalistic views of the sabbath, took time out to rest and experience the depths of God's creative love. Luke 4:31–44 describes a day in the life of Jesus. Each moment of Jesus's day was filled to the brim with service and teaching: healing the demon-possessed, dining with friends, healing the sick, teaching at the synagogue. But, as the next day began Jesus "departed and went into a lonely place"(Luke 4:42).

The sabbath provides us with an opportunity to find a quiet and solitary place for prayer and reflection. For modern persons, the sabbath may not best be observed in terms of a specific day of the week. Because of my Sunday responsibilities at the university chapel and the busy spirit of Saturdays often filled with weddings and university events, I typically take Friday as my personal sabbath for rest, re-creation, and family time. "Sabbath time" is an attitude toward life. Those who observe the sabbath realize that the world can go on without them. They perceive their lives as part of a larger story—the story of God's presence in universal and human history. In light of eternity, the individual tasks and moments of life take on a new perspective, for they are connected with God's presence in all times and places. Time, like our bodies, becomes a temple or sanctuary wherein we encounter the holy.

Spiritual guide Tilden Edwards counsels persons to practice "sabbath moments" throughout the week—momentary withdrawals from doing and achieving in order to reconnect with God, our deepest selves, and those around us.[14] In so doing, we discover the meaning of Abraham Heschel's words: "the Sabbath surrounds you wherever you go."[15]

For some persons, such as working parents of newborns or persons working long hours (medical residents or those in other demanding positions), a literal sabbath day may not be possible. Instead of feeling guilty about what we cannot do, we can gracefully commit ourselves to what we can do to reduce stress and nurture our spiritual lives. We can take a sabbath each day, through moments of quiet and devotional reading. We can also take a momentary sabbath—as we sit at a traffic light, when the phone rings, or at the tolling of a nearby church bell—by saying brief prayers or breathing quietly the spirit of God. In my own busy days at the university, I try to practice the discipline of a brief prayer for guidance and peace whenever the phone rings, the college bell tolls, or I hear a knock at my door. I am conscious of my own tendency to become so wrapped up in my work that any break becomes a nuisance or threat to the task at hand. I am amazed how different my attitude becomes when I turn to prayer rather than annoyance, in relationship to the many unplanned interruptions of my day.

In practicing sabbath time, we realize that God's presence is ubiquitous. We cannot escape God's care spatially or temporally. We can trust God to provide for our deepest needs even as we plan for the future. We can relax because the ultimate issues of our lives find their meaning, purpose, and fruition in God's hands. Truly, our times are in God's hands.[16]

2. *Meditation for spirituality and stress reduction.* The disciplines of daily meditation, prayer, and spiritual reading create a sabbath amid everyday life. Recently, it has been discovered that prayer and meditation have physiological as well as spiritual benefits. In the next chapter, I will focus on the power of prayer. In the following paragraphs, I consider two forms of meditation—the "relaxation response" of Herbert Benson and "centering prayer" as taught by Basil Pennington.

According to Herbert Benson, most persons in modern societies are unconscious victims of the "fight or flight" response. Long ago, the "fight or flight" response was necessary for human survival. Confronted by a dangerous beast or an enemy, it was essential that the body mobilize itself quickly by increasing the blood pressure, heart rate, rate of breathing, flow of blood to the muscles, and metabolism. Persons discharged this physiological rush through running, fighting, and climbing. Today, there are few saber-toothed tigers in our midst. But, persons still feel themselves at risk and the body mobilizes itself to respond to the imagined or real threats to its well-being. For example, when I imagine an upcoming conflict situation or obsess on a less than perfect encounter with a friend or associate, I also experience my heartbeat and breath quickening. Unfortunately, the stresses and pressures of life that lead to the "fight or flight" response are seldom discharged in the course of everyday life. Chronic and repeated experiences of the "fight or flight" response wear down the body and may lead to heart disease, stroke, or the breakdown of the immune system.

There is, however, an antidote to the "fight or flight" response. This easy-to-learn antidote is the "relaxation response." In contrast to the "fight or flight response," the relaxation response leads to an involuntary reduction in the sympathetic system and decreases the body's oxygen consumption, metabolism, heartbeat, and blood pressure.[17] While we cannot change the nature of the external stresses of modern life, we can, Benson believes, "prevent some of the negative side effects through the relaxation response."[18]

For the most beneficial results, the relaxation response should be practiced twice a day for 15-20 minutes at a time. In its simplicity, the relaxation response can be learned by virtually everyone. Its four elements are: 1) a quiet environment, 2) a mental device, such as a word or phrase which is repeated in a specific fashion over and over again, 3) a receptive and non-judgmental attitude toward thoughts that emerge, 4) a comfortable position.

Recently, Benson has recognized the importance of the religious dimension for the effectiveness of the relaxation response. While merely repeating a secular word will lower one's metabolism and reverse the effects of stressful living, the addition of a religious context combines the impact of the relaxation response with the placebo effect. Put simply, the placebo effect is the impact of our beliefs on our physiology. If we believe a drug has certain positive side effects (such as decrease of pain or increased mobility), our body tends to exhibit these effects even if the medication is chemically inert. Religious beliefs have the same impact, Benson asserts.

The "faith factor" combines the relaxation response with one's religious beliefs. Benson contends that the "faith factor" can relieve headaches and angina pectoris pain, decrease blood pressure, enhance cancer therapy, respond to backaches, and reduce overall stress.[19] Benson asserts that "if you truly believe in your philosophy or religious faith—if you are committed, mind and soul, to your world view—you may be capable of achieving remarkable feats of mind and body that many only speculate about."[20] Religious faith, described in terms of the placebo effect, is enough to change our physiology: in 75% of medical situations, our beliefs can play a major role in healing physical ills.[21]

While Christians believe that connecting with God in prayer and meditation is more than a placebo, they can, nevertheless, profit by joining their beliefs and personal prayers with a simple meditative technique such as the relaxation response. Benson asserts that the heart of this approach is the choice of a meaningful word that reflects one's deepest spiritual beliefs. For example, Christians might choose a phrase from the Lord's Prayer ("thy will be done"), or Psalm 23 ("the Lord is my shepherd"), or a traditional prayer such as the "Jesus prayer" (Lord, have mercy upon me, a sinner). They might simply choose a meaningful word to repeat over and over again such as "Jesus," "God," "love," "spirit," or "peace." This spiritual elaboration of the relaxation response contains the following elements: 1) the choice of a meaningful word or symbol, 2) a comfortable position, 3) closing one's eyes, 4) relaxing one's mind, 5) becoming aware of breathing, 6) maintaining a passive and receptive attitude.

The regular use of this spiritual version of the relaxation response reconnects and restores our relationship with our deepest self and with God. When reconnected with the vine, the vitality of God's innate healing presence refreshes one's whole being and renews one's body and spirit.

Similar to Benson's relaxation response is "centering prayer" as taught by Catholic monk Basil Pennington. Centering prayer is the recovery of the ancient monastic practice of reciting a word or phrase as part of one's spiritual discipline. Rather than practicing Hindu forms of meditation, such as transcendental meditation, or secular forms of meditation (the initial forms of the relaxation response, for example), Christians will benefit from using a prayer technique grounded in their own faith tradition. In its simplicity, centering prayer can be learned by virtually anyone. It involves simply:

1) Taking a moment to relax in a comfortable position.

2) Opening oneself in faith and love to God's presence in the center of one's being.

3) Focusing on a "love word" (for example, God, Jesus, light, or love).

4) Bringing oneself gently and without judgment back to the love word, whenever the mind wanders.

5) Concluding with the Lord's Prayer.[22]

I have used forms of transcendental meditation, the relaxation response, and centering prayer for over 25 years and have taught versions of centering prayer for nearly 20 years. I have found that these simple techniques bring immediate peace and stress reduction to myself and others. When practiced regularly as part of one's spiritual disciplines, they enhance personal creativity and make the Scriptures come alive in unexpected and insightful ways. If, indeed, the spirit of God is constantly speaking through us, centering prayer and the spiritual use of the relaxation response enable us to enhance our conscious and unconscious encounter with the spirit and effortlessly access the ever-present healing power of God. Resting in God, we no longer need to be as anxious about our lives. Calm descends upon our bodies and spirits when we remember that God's peace is always with us.

While these meditative prayers are most effective when we sit in meditation for fifteen minutes or more, I have found that momentary focus on one's prayer word also can bring a sense of peace and centeredness. Since much of our stress is a form of stimulus-response, we can teach our minds to become peaceful merely by repeating our prayer word as we take a test, go to a meeting, or prepare for a difficult conversation. I often take a few deep breaths and imagine God's light flooding my being before teaching, speaking, or negotiating a problematic situation. Almost always, I begin to feel less anxious and more in tune with God's will in the situation.

3. *Living by our affirmations.* The biblical tradition asserts that words are creative and powerful. God creates the universe by the Word and the Word of God is the principle of both order and salvation. Persons' names were not accidental in the ancient world. A change in one's name indicated a change in one's self-awareness and relationship—Jacob the "trickster" is renamed Israel, the "one who contends with God and humankind and prevails" after his encounter with God at the stream of Jabbok; Saul is renamed Paul following his encounter with the risen Lord. In recent years, feminist the-

ologians have reminded us that words about God and humankind can exclude and dehumanize as well as include and uplift.

In the medical field, psychoneuroimmunologists and researchers have recognized that the word is a chemical event whose impact is omnipresent in our body, mind, and emotions. From the perspective of the organic and relational understanding of human existence, all aspects of our lives are shaped by the language we use. Words can imprison or liberate, they can cure or they can harm.

Sadly, most of the language we grow up with is negative in tone. As children, words such as "don't," "can't," "no," and "stop" fill our consciousness and shape our perception of ourselves and the world. The words we hear in childhood and throughout our lives enter our unconscious and condition our behavior and responses to life's challenges. When I was a child, I heard the message that I was not a good artist. Only recently have I taken the chance to draw more than stick figures. Other persons hear and internalize messages such as "you will never be successful," "you are powerless to change your life," "the world is indifferent to your needs," "other people cannot be trusted," or "you are not worthy of love." The words we use have an emotional content and a physiological impact. The unconscious language we live by may be a matter of life and death, as studies of Type A personalities and persons with cancer suggest.

The Christian vision of reality, however, claims that persons can be transformed and that the "new creation" brought about by God's grace liberates us from past memories, habits, and ways of interpreting our lives. A holistic vision of salvation asserts that God is able to transform and is constantly seeking to heal even those things about which we are unconscious.

Recently, motivation coaches and psychologists have affirmed the importance of "self talk" in personal transformation. According to motivational speaker Shad Helmstetter, "our conscious thoughts and words are reflections of the unconscious programs that create them."[23] When we are unaware of our unconscious scripts and self talk, we become victims of past conditioning, which limits our creativity and joy of life. Helmstetter asserts that one's physical well-being depends on consciously redirecting one's thoughts and words, since "any input the brain receives affects you both physically and mentally."[24]

Freedom and creativity blossom when we take control of the language of our lives. "What we do is determined by the programming we receive; if we want to change what happens next, we have to change the programming."[25] By repeating positive affirmations on a regular basis, we replace negative self talk with consciously chosen positive self talk. Since the unconscious cannot distinguish between internal and external language, it accepts the directions we consciously give it, and these directions are eventually reflected in our attitudes, lifestyle, health, and relationships.

The use of affirmations and positive self talk has been helpful in responding to the diagnosis of cancer. Many inaccurate myths surround cancer and its treatment. O. Carl Simonton has identified three culturally and medically conditioned myths about cancer: 1) cancer is synonymous with death, 2) cancer is something that strikes from without and there is little a person can do to control it, 3) treatment is always drastic and has undesirable side effects.[26] Simonton's program for treating cancer involves a renewing of the mind and a challenging of cancer myths as well as medical care. Simonton's patients are invited to visualize as well as intellectually recognize that cancer cells are not omnipotent as the cancer myths suggest, but weak and confused in comparison to the strength and focus of the immune system; that each person has a responsibility for choosing health or illness; and that the treatment is an ally and friend on the road to recovery. By the use of affirmations one moves from being a victim to being an agent of one's own healing process. Jerry Jampolsky, a psychiatrist well known for his work with children with cancer, concurs with the Simonton approach: the use of affirmations transforms the mind from a dysfunctional to a creative belief system. In so doing, we are liberated from false self-images and perceptions of our limitations to a true understanding of our self and its power.

Christians are called to live by their affirmations. Recognizing that stress, hopelessness, and disconnectedness arise from the perception of an indifferent and unfriendly world, Christians are challenged to take the words of their faith seriously and repeat them as antidotes to the negativity of the world. Every time a person declares one of the ecumenical creeds of the church—the Apostles' or Nicene Creed—they are affirming a distinctively creative and life-supporting worldview. "I believe in God the Father Almighty, maker of heaven and earth" proclaims that we live in a personal and benevolent universe. To speak of God as the mighty creator and affirm God's redemptive love is to relativize all the threats of this world and place them in the context of God's eternal care. To affirm that I believe in "the communion of saints, the forgiveness of sins, the resurrection of the body, and life everlasting" is to claim that my life is in God's hands and that I am no longer controlled by the hands of the clock, a medical diagnosis, or other persons' concepts of me. To affirm the "communion of saints" is to ground myself in a world of creative and healing relationships. In light of a holistic understanding of the resurrection of the body, each day is a unique gift full of promise and adventure because it shares in God's eternity.

Christian faith affirms that the word is made flesh in healing encounters and moments of personal transformation. Our use of healing affirmations "embodies" the faith we affirm and enables us to respond creatively to life's crises. In my own spiritual discipline, I regularly use affirmations both for prevention and transformation. The following biblical affirmations have been pivotal in my own spiritual journey:

> I can do all things through Christ who strengthens me.
> Nothing can separate me from the love of God.
> You are the light of the world.
> Do not be afraid, for I have redeemed you.
> Not I but Christ within me.
> My body is the temple of God.
> My faith is making me whole.
> Christ within me, the hope of glorious things to come.
> God's light shines in me.
> My God shall supply your every need.
> Whether we live or die, we belong to God.
> All things work together for good for those who love God.
> In all things, we are more than conquerors.
> My times are in God's hands.

Other non-scriptural Christian affirmations, grounded in the biblical tradition, include:

> Through God's grace, I am healthy and strong.
> Through God's grace, I respond to problems creatively.
> I am healed in body, mind, and spirit.
> God is constantly giving me new and creative ideas for God's glory and my neighbor's welfare.
> My illness is in God's hands.
> God is giving me the resources to be victorious.
> Through God's grace, I have enough time.
> God's peace is mine.
> In Christ, I have all the time, money, and energy to succeed, flourish, and serve God.

Through the use of affirmations, we open to God's new creation. We move from a world based on fear, hopelessness, unforgiveness, and isolation, to a world abundant in possibility, love, friendship, and healing. A new vision of reality awakens a new self and a new relationship with God. The impact of such transformation is physiological as well as spiritual. While the use of affirmations or any spiritual discipline does not insure healing or deliverance from life's problems, affirmative living enables us to see our lives, problems, illness, and eventual death in a larger, more supportive perspective. Our negative emotions and thoughts, our physical pain and aging, are no longer the *only* reality but merely one aspect of a multidimensional world. As we open to an affirmative and faith-filled image of our lives and God's presence within them, we discover that even pain and death need not hinder our spiritual growth, our care for others, and our relationship to God.

d) Imagination and healing. The prophet proclaims that "without a vision, the people perish." Current medical studies have affirmed the significance of imagination in the promotion of physical well-being. In speaking of the importance of visualization and imagination, Robert Ader, one of the pioneers in the field of psychoneuroimmunology, asserts "the connection between mind/emotion, central nervous system, the autonomic nervous system, and the immune system."[27] As most of us know from experience, the "fight or flight" response can be elicited merely by fantasy or a memory. Our visions, dreams, and fantasies give direction and vividness to our lives. But they do not end in our minds. A holistic vision of human existence asserts that the imagination is physiological as well as psychological. Medical research has found that the use of imagination and visualization not only engenders optimism, peace of mind, and hope but also increases the number of circulating white blood cells, increases immune function, and enhances the production of helper T-cells.

Persons who used imagery in conjunction with surgical procedures have been found to need less time for recuperation in the hospital.[28]

In his pioneering work with visualization and imagination, O. Carl Simonton uses images such as Pac Man, Star Wars, radiant streams of light, and bullets to enhance the effectiveness of radiation and chemical therapy.

Simonton's use of imagery is reflected in the following case study of his treatment of a sixty-one-year-old man with throat cancer:

> Next, Carl asked him to picture his treatment, radiation therapy, as consisting of millions of tiny bullets of energy that would hit all the cells, both normal and cancerous, in their path. Because the cancer cells were weaker and more confused, they would not be able to repair the damage... and so the normal cells would remain healthy while the cancer cells would die.
>
> Carl asked the patient to form a mental picture of the last and most important step—his body's white blood cells coming in, swarming over the cancer cells, picking up and carrying off the dead and dying ones, flushing them off his body through his liver and kidneys. In his mind's eye he was to visualize the cancer decreasing in size and his health returning to normal.[29]

Simonton claims that patients using imagery have recovered more fully and with fewer side effects than the typical cancer patient. At the very least, such imagery reframes the treatment as an ally and cancer as weak, enabling the patient to become an actor rather a victim.

Imagination is at the center of biblical spirituality. Walter Brueggeman, in his *Prophetic Imagination*, sees one of the tasks of prophetic spirituality as presenting an alternative vision to the culture's ways of death and injustice. In the area of health, the imagination serves a similar purpose—it invites personal transformation by presenting an alternative vision to painful memories, to feelings of victimization and stress, and to self-imposed limitations. The use of creative imagination is our invitation to claim the power of God and healing relationships in a world that often nurtures isolation and loneliness.

Imagination was central to the parables of Jesus. The parables challenge our usual way of looking at reality—the Samaritan is the "hero," the prodigal son is welcomed home, a tiny seed quietly grows into the greatest of bushes. Jesus' ministry was an experiment in imagination. Jesus saw the divine in its most hidden disguises—he saw a rock in the impetuous Peter, a saint in a prostitute, an evangelist in a dishonest tax collector.

In the tradition of spiritual direction, *The Spiritual Exercises* of Ignatius of Loyola, the spiritual father of the Society of Jesus (Jesuits), employ the imagination as means of experiencing God's grace through the Scriptures. As the Scripture is read, one is invited to place oneself within the story: to observe the annunciation and the birth of Jesus; to experience the tragic consequence of original sin; to participate in the Last Supper; and to witness the death and resurrection.[30] The Bible is not merely a book of words, but a collection of lively images. The reader is challenged to become a participant in the biblical witness and to find her or his place in God's ongoing revelation in human existence.

While "creative visualization" has been central to many new age spiritual disciplines, it has also been appropriated by Christian healers. Ruth Carter Stapleton utilized imagery as a means of healing painful memories. Stapleton found that the healing of memories often led to new vitality and physical health among those she prayed with. If, as Simonton and Lawrence LeShan suggest, the emotional wounds of childhood can predispose certain people toward cancer, then the healing of memories may constitute a significant preventative measure. According to Stapleton, "when we pray for inner healing, we are really asking Jesus to walk into the dark places of our lives and bring healing to the distressing and painful memories of the past."[31] Stapleton believes that through the use of faith-imagination, "the mind fills the emotional space occupied by a negative thought or memory with a new, more powerful, positive image or thought."[32] Negative memories are replaced by a God-inspired reconstruction of these memories.

Stapleton's techniques are Christ-centered. To enable one to forgive an offense, she is invited to experience Christ's love flow into the offender as she seeks to forgive them.[33] In dealing with a painful memory, we are invited to imagine Jesus moving back into our lives with us, loving the wounded child, and healing the wounded child by giving him the love he wished a parent might have given. When a painful memory surfaces, Stapleton counsels that we go back to the memory of the most deeply felt pain. As the situation is recalled in all its emotional pain, one is called to image Jesus as one's companion in that situation and then ask Jesus to respond to you in the way that was most needed at the time. In response to a young man who was afraid of the dark, Stapleton counseled "to imagine that just outside the door Jesus is waiting for you" and that Jesus would walk with him in the darkness.[34] In the spirit of her evangelical faith, Stapleton asserts that Jesus is the Lord of all things—the imagination, the unconscious, and the repressed memory. Positive imagination brings health and healing because it places us within the divine flow.

In my own work, I employ imagination for stress reduction and personal healing. I invite persons experiencing great stress to take a few minutes to relax, to observe their bodies and their breath, and then to see themselves in a beautiful and peaceful place with Jesus as their companion. As they sit together, I invite them to share their anxiety with Jesus, to listen to Jesus' response, and then ask Jesus to bear their burden with them. Another visualization I often use involves experiencing the burden of a heavy backpack as one walks up a mountain path, and then meeting a stranger who asks to carry the pack. The backpack is filled with all one's tasks and worries. This unknown stranger is Jesus, who carries our burdens when they are too great for ourselves.

I have often used the "storm at sea" as a response to stress. I invite persons to be among Jesus' disciples as they set off across the Sea of Galilee, to experience the brightness of the sun, and then the fear brought on by a sudden storm. I ask the persons, then, to reflect on the storms in their lives. Amid the personal storms and the storm at sea, I invite them to remember that Jesus is with them in the boat, and to experience the peace that comes from experiencing Jesus' companionship.

For persons struggling to experience personal healing, I often employ the story of the man at the pool of Bethesda. I invite them to hear Jesus ask them, "do you want to be healed?" and, then, after reflecting on the impediments to healing in their lives, respond to Jesus' command, "stand up, take your bed, and walk."

A healing visualization I often employ in my own self-healing involves the invocation of God's light. I believe that in many illnesses, there is a pivotal moment where our choice for health can prevent any further symptoms. When I feel myself coming down with a cold or the flu, I take time to center down, find a comfortable place, and notice my breath. As I breathe, I image a golden healing light, filling my body—my mind, my circulatory system, my immune system, my cells—in its entirety, with special focus on the area of disease. This visualization has often proved effective in preventing or alleviating the symptoms of a potential illness.

In visualization, just as in affirmations, sabbath time, and meditation, we are called to align ourselves with God's healing presence as it is manifest in our bodies and minds. Visualization, like the other practices, is grounded in the recognition of both the negative realities we face and the positive power of God.

IV. Concluding Remarks

As we open ourselves to the disciplines of spiritual transformation, we discover that God's power is greater than our problems. These disciplines work precisely because they unite our fears and stresses with the omnipresent healing love of God as it flows through our bodies, our emotions and thoughts, the events, and the apparently random encounters with other seekers. The external stresses will not go away. We may also find ourselves troubled by internal forms of stress—painful memories, feelings of depression, scarcity, and hopelessness. But, when we connect with God's healing power, we become a new creation, and though memories of the past remain and hopelessness may still plague us, they will not overwhelm us. We will no longer be victims of our emotions, the ticking clock, or others' expectations, for we will have discovered that we are connected with God's grace and this is sufficient for us.

Questions for Reflection and Discussion

1) How would you assess your current level of stress? What events or thoughts create stress in your life?

2) Do you take time out to relax and re-create? What are the benefits of such mini-sabbaths?

3) How do you respond to the idea of a sabbath? How does this reflect your own theological perspective?

4) What is your experience of prayer and meditation? Do

you think we can connect with God in times of quiet as well as spoken prayer?

5) What positive or negative affirmations characterize your personal worldview and self-perception?

6) What biblical affirmations would be most helpful to you now?

7) What is your response to the use of affirmations for spiritual growth or health enhancement? What biblical images are most powerful in your experience?

Chapter Four

Prayer in an Age of Science and Medicine

I. Exploring the Power of Prayer

Prayer has become fashionable in medical circles these days. Physicians who believe in the power of prayer are spotlighted in popular magazines and television talk shows. In an age of technological wonders and medical miracles, the growing interest in the power of prayer is both surprising and understandable. Physicians and patients alike have realized that the spiritual realm has an impact on many of the physical and emotional issues that are beyond the scope of our technological expertise. Indeed, unearthing the mysteries of the power of prayer may become the next frontier of medical research.

Spirituality and religious commitment, which had been banished from the medical world for centuries as unscientific, useless, and superstitious, are now being viewed as essential to physical and mental health. The National Institute of Healthcare Research (NIHR) has recently compiled a four-volume study of medical research relating to the "faith factor," or the role of spirituality, faith, and religious commitment in promoting good health. Dr. Dale Matthews, a professor of Internal Medicine at Georgetown University and one of the authors of the NIHR study, has become well known for his willingness to pray with his patients. His example is being emulated in many examination rooms every day. Dr. Deepak Chopra's books on the relationship of Hindu spirituality, ayurvedic medicine, and health have made the best-seller lists. Dr. Larry Dossey has recently written of his own interest in prayer and health and has asserted that a physician who believes in the power of prayer, but does not utilize it for the welfare of her or his patients, may be in some way negligent in their treatment.[1]

Physicians are discovering what their more religious patients have always known—that prayer makes a difference and that difference may be a matter of life and death. Recently, Dr. Randolph Byrd, a San Francisco physician, studied 393 coronary care patients at San Francisco General Hospital. Of the 393 patients, 192 were regularly prayed for by name by a group of evangelical Christians, while the other 201, the "control group" in this double-blind study, were not prayed for by the prayer group. While the results deserve both scientific and theological scrutiny, they are impressive, to say the least. Byrd found that those prayed for required five times fewer antibiotics, experienced three times fewer medical complications, and did not require breathing tubes (compared to twelve in the control group.)[2] Some commentators have joyfully noted that praying to the Judeo-Christian God may enhance health and should be placed on the medical protocols of all coronary care units! Other studies have examined the effects of prayer at a distance on plants and the effectiveness of certain styles of prayer. Although it has been found that prayer universally makes a difference, studies have also indicated that nondirected ("thy will be done") prayers may be more effective than directed prayers. Directed or goal-oriented prayers seem, however, to be more effective than ritualized prayers, recited from prayer books or memory.

While Christians should be pleased that the scientific world is recognizing the power of prayer, it is important that we do not judge prayer by the standards of science or cost-benefit analysis. Prayer is not just another technological fix, like antibiotics, genetic screening, or bypass surgery. If the practice of prayer is to make a positive difference in the long run to physicians, patients, and communities of faith, then prayer must be understood in the context of a proper theological, spiritual, and practical perspective. While a healthy world-view, grounded in good theology, is a contributing factor in the health of mind, body, and spirit, a dysfunctional or naive theological position may lead to the guilt and self-blame that open the door to illness.

A healthy vision of prayer must avoid two equally danger-ous extremes: impotence (the belief that persons have no power to determine their fate and that prayer makes absolute-ly no difference in our well-being or the well-being of others) and omnipotence (the belief that persons can "name it and claim it" or "create their own realities" and, thus, control real-ity by their prayers). A healthy vision of prayer must avoid using the recent medical findings in such a way that prayer becomes identified as a magic bullet or technological fix, whose results are always predictable and whose practice can be encouraged independent of a living relationship with God. To date, no scientific study of prayer can assess the role of God in responding to our prayers; nor is one likely to be found!

Ironically, a healthy vision of prayer depends as much on a theology of "unanswered prayer" as it does on a theological understanding of "answered" prayer. Prayer is not magic or the manipulation of a higher power; it is openness to God's dynamic and surprising presence in our lives and in the world. Prayer is an essential factor in the well-being of the "temple of God." In this chapter, we will explore both the theological and practical implications of prayer in a scientific age. In the next chapter, we will reflect on a theological understanding of the miraculous. My goal is simply to promote healthy and life-supporting images and practices of prayer and theologically grounded understandings of the role of God in human life.

One of the mysteries of prayer is the difficulty we have defining it. At the very least, prayer can be understood in terms of a person's openness to God's presence in her or his life. But, in practice, this openness takes many forms, ranging from cries for help to "a power greater than ourselves," to listening for God's voice in silence and experiencing God as an intimate companion. However we understand it, prayer connects us with the "body of Christ" and awakens us to the dynamic energy of "the vine" of which we are branches.

II. Prayer in the Biblical Tradition

The scriptural tradition is an essential resource for any Christian understanding of the practice of prayer. In its role as one of Christianity's primary resources for understanding the divine-human relationship, Scripture in its many voices provides a compelling and influential vision of health and illness. The biblical witness, especially among the prophets and Jesus of Nazareth, affirms a holistic vision of prayer, health, and healing. Although Christians cannot read Scripture naively or in a piecemeal fashion or neglect the fact that there is typically no one biblical position on the most significant issues of life and human destiny, the biblical witness to God's presence in human life still inspires persons to open their lives to the deeper healing dimensions of reality. Scripture proclaims that God seeks healing and liberation from all that oppresses humankind, be it spiritual, physical, or political in nature.

Virtually every prayer form found in the Western world can be traced to the scriptural witness. Quaker meditation and silent prayer can be traced to the words of Psalm 46, "be still and know that I am God." The use of mantras, or words of spiritual focus characteristic of centering prayer, is rooted in Paul's admonition to "pray without ceasing" (1 Thessalonians 5:17). Jesus' use of parables invites persons to explore the visualization techniques characteristic of Ignatian spirituality and contemporary guided meditation. Jesus' invitation to "ask, seek, and knock," recorded in the Sermon on the Mount (Matthew 7:7), inspires prayers of petition and intercession to a God who hears and responds to our deepest needs.

At the heart of the Christian understanding of prayer is the image of God as "abba," as the Father or Parent of all creation. Prayer is a possibility precisely because God has a personal and intimate relationship with each creature. The gospel proclamation, "for God so loved the world that he gave his only begotten Son" (John 3:16), is a personal address to everyone that God loves you and God wants you to experience salvation or wholeness in this life and the next. Paul's affirmation that the "Spirit intercedes for us in sighs too deep for words" (Romans 8:26) is a reminder that God addresses us from within our own spirits in terms of our deepest desires. This address is intensely personal in nature as it permeates both the conscious and unconscious mind.

The gospel proclaims that God is on our side and that God desires our well-being. The hallmark of Jesus' ministry is his embodiment of God's desire that all might have "abundant life" (John 10:10). Although some biblical passages imply that illness is the result of divine punishment or a linear calculus of rewards and punishment (John 9:1–4), the ministry of Jesus points to an entirely different attitude toward health and illness. Although our beliefs, actions, and life-style may contribute to spiritual, emotional, and physical illness, these negative results are not caused by God. God's primary motivation is that the sick be healed and the healthy continue to flourish.

As we will see more clearly in the chapter on healing and miracles, the biblical tradition affirms that faith is a factor in health and healing. To those who would doubt the power of God in the lives of the faithful, Jesus proclaims that "if you have faith the size of a mustard seed, you will say to this mountain, 'move from here to there,' and it will move, and nothing will be impossible for you" (Matthew 17:20). When we align ourselves with the will of God, coincidences and acts of power, otherwise known as miracles, come to pass.

III. Power or Placebo?

Despite the biblical witness to the power of prayer, we still must ask, "is the power of prayer merely a placebo, the physiological response to one's belief system, or does it truly reflect the divine-human encounter?" This question has surfaced as a result of the fact that prayer seems to be effective regardless of one's religious tradition or theological perspective. While medical research cannot answer this question, recent studies on the positive role of religious behavior and belief in health point to a new frontier in the relationship of spirituality and health care.

The positive impact of religious commitment and life-style is obvious from the standpoint of recent medical research. Belonging to a church and praying regularly may be as effective as exercise or diet in longevity and good health. Countless examples of the intersection of religion and health are found in the massive NIHR study of the role of religion in health. One study, for example, indicates that religious belief leads to less death anxiety.[3] It is easy to assume that lower anxiety will decrease blood pressure and wear and tear on the body, and thus increase overall well-being and longevity. Seventh Day Adventists, whose faith is reflected in a healthy diet, live longer and healthier lives than other groups.[4]

Religious activity has not only been identified with longevity, it has also been connected with greater happiness.[5] While scientists cannot identify the reasons why church activity enhances health, studies indicate that regular church attendance leads to lower blood pressure and fewer incidences of certain types of ailments.[6] In its commentary on Randolph Byrd's previously cited study of coronary patients at San Francisco General Hospital, the NIHR document asks, "should all patients in all coronary care units throughout the world have intercessory prayer to the Judeo-Christian God ordered by their attending doctor?"[7] In a recent lecture, physician Dale Matthews notes that the physician's advice to pray may be as beneficial as the counsel to exercise or wear a seat belt.

Such jubilant comments are dampened by Larry Dossey's statement that among psychic healers, including some Christians, prayer seems to be only 20% effective. Further, prayer seems to be more effective in addressing certain ailments than others. Seldom, except in the context of the often grandiose and theatrical claims of television healers, do we hear of new limbs being grown, the blind receiving sight, or final stage cancers being cured. Prayer seems to be most effective in those specifically mind-spirit-emotion-body ailments, where trust, peace, and confidence make the difference between life and death. Nevertheless, for those who suffer from chronic illness, being among the 20% who find healing is the difference between hope and hopelessness.

In a world in which quantum physics and ecological/relational thinking have altered the way we envision the universe, we must also understand prayer in terms of new images and practices. Prayer must be seen in terms of an ecology of dynamic interrelationships. Linear cause and effect understandings of prayer lead to feelings of impotence and omnipotence insofar as they place the entire responsibility of prayer on the efforts of the pray-er herself or on the power of God alone. What is needed today is a theology of prayer that addresses both "successes" and "failures" in our prayer lives and encourages persons to take the practice of prayer seriously in their own health and the health of their loved ones.

IV. A Theology of Prayer

Each day, millions of persons take a few moments for a time of prayer. For some, it is an affirmation about God's goodness and their own potential at the beginning of the day. For others, a scriptural proclamation, "this is the day the Lord has made, I will rejoice and be glad in it," is a call to dwell in awareness of God's goodness throughout the day. As a couple joins hands in marriage, the priest or pastor and congregation bow in prayer and take time to bless them for their journey ahead. In a small group on campus or in the neighborhood, persons share prayer concerns and pause for an extended time of intercession and petition. This morning, I have already prayed briefly with a student who is "stressed out" over an upcoming exam and a coworker who is in the university hospital. Such pastoral experiences are hardly unusual and are not reserved to the ordained ministry. Even an atheist may visit a church after a friend dies, looking for someone beyond the human realm to listen or someone upon whom to shower her anger and grief. In times of national mourning or crisis, the President calls for a moment of silent prayer and concludes with words such as "God bless the United States of America."

Prayer is universal in time, place, and content. Some form of prayer is articulated in every religion and culture. Even our commonplace greetings and farewells—"hello" and "good bye"—have their origins in the personal blessings—"health to you" and "God be with you."

Although prayer is universally practiced in one form or

another, even by those who don't claim to be religious, prayer still remains a mystery to believer and agnostic alike. The recent medical studies on the power of prayer have not demystified it. In fact, scientific studies may even add to the mystery of prayer. Prayer is unpredictable in its results and no one technique seems to fit all persons or occasions. The prayer of one faithful person may move mountains, while a whole nation's prayer may not avert catastrophe. Further, in times of personal, political, or international conflict, the prayers of the faithful may contradict one another. Fervent prayers may be given, asking God to end the national erosion of the sanctity of life, while equally fervent prayers may be given with the hope that our nation will enact laws that provide a painless method for ending the suffering of the terminally ill.

No doubt, from the perspective of the secular scientist and the closed systems of research, prayer is no more than a placebo. Our beliefs, optimism, and confidence in a reality beyond ourselves shape our perception of the world and the events of our lives. Without a doubt, feelings of optimism and interconnectedness with life influence our physical health. But most pray-ers believe prayer to be more than "self-talk" or "positive thinking." Prayer is an encounter with the ultimate reality, the living and personal God. It is the experience of connectedness with the "true vine," a divine power much greater and wiser than ourselves.

Even if prayer is no more than a focused version of the relaxation response, the "faith factor" at the heart of prayer plays a role in physical and spiritual transformation. What is astonishing to believer and agnostic alike is the fact that prayer often makes a difference regardless of our piety or the conformation of our beliefs with the nature of the one true God. (Remember the example of the infidel's frantic prayer being answered, while the saint dies of cancer.) Prayer connects us with an "open system" in which unexpected events are the norm. As a noted minister confessed, "when I pray, coincidences happen." Prayer, like grace, loses its meaning when it is no longer surprising.

Even if the scientist cannot explicitly discover God's presence in the recent studies that point to the power of prayer, the reality of prayer and its positive impact on our spiritual, emotional, and physical health point to a bias in the universe and in our bodies. The universe aims at order, well-being, and abundant life. Trust and love are transformative of oneself and others, even when such love is prayerfully expressed from a distance. The fact that the scientist cannot find God through the usual practice of the scientific method, however, is no argument against God's existence or the divine-human encounter in prayerful moments. To think that our knowledge determines the nature of reality itself is the height of intellectual arrogance and pride. Faith itself may give persons, as the mystics claim, a form of perception beyond normal sense perception. The higher sense perception characteristic of deep prayer enables persons to encounter the higher dimensions of reality, traditionally related to God. As we ponder the recent medical findings on the power of prayer in the context of the mystical tradition and contemporary quantum physics, we must update our spiritual geography even as we update our scientific and medical maps of the world.

To the believer, prayer has always been more than a placebo, or something merely to give us courage in difficult times. Prayer taps into the most basic power of the universe—the power of God. Although we do not know how prayer affects God or the exact nature of the divine response to prayer, prayers believe that God is responsive to the deepest desires of the human heart.

Our desire to pray is grounded in the faith that God is loving and that God will provide for our deepest needs.

The pluralism of our time reminds us that there is no consensus on the nature of ultimate reality. New agers have challenged the notion of a personal God, while feminists have contested the traditional Western images of God as patriarchal and hierarchical. Although no one vision of God expresses the wholeness of God's nature, it is equally clear that some images of God encourage prayerful relationship and basic trust while others make the practice of prayer a virtual impossibility. If the image of the body of Christ is a significant metaphor for the relationship of God and the world and God's presence in human life, then certain images of prayer can be affirmed as healthy and life-supporting, while others can be disregarded as ineffective or dysfunctional. In the next few paragraphs, we will explore the nature of prayer as a dynamic process in the body of Christ and articulate a healthy vision of the practice of prayer. I will conclude this chapter with a reflection on the "practice of the presence of God" as it relates in a practical manner to our prayer lives and our health.

Most pray-ers understand prayer in terms of communication or relationship with God. The God who answers prayers is not distant, aloof, or only occasionally active in the world; God is dynamic, living, creative, and personal. In the language of interpersonal relationships, God listens, mirrors, and responds to our deepest needs. Jesus' use of the word "abba" or "daddy" to describe God's relationship to humankind points to the intimacy of the one who speaks and the one who listens. God loves the world and God loves me! As an early Church Father once proclaimed, "God is the circle whose center is everywhere and whose circumference is nowhere."

The image of the body of Christ reinforces the intimacy between God and each creature. When we understand the image of the body of Christ in psychosomatic or holistic terms, then we can compare the relationship of God and creation, parts and whole, to the mind-body relationship. Psychosomatic medicine maintains that the mind is omnipresent in the body and that the body is constantly influencing the mind. There is no clear boundary between mind and body, nor is there a distinct boundary between God and the world. The mind alters the body, within limits imposed by the environment and one's physical condition, by acting on the body in terms of challenges, feelings, and ideals, and the "divine circle whose center is everywhere" *centers* itself on each and every part of the "body."

Paul's notion of "Christ in me" is not merely a spiritual or moral platitude; it is a recognition of the reality that Christ is present in the depths of the human spirit and the body, even when Christ is not affirmed or recognized. Further, Paul's affirmation that the spirit speaks within us in "sighs too deep for words" suggests that God is always active in the deepest levels of our experience, both spiritual and physical. Indeed, the incarnation and the eucharist proclaim that we cannot fully know God apart from the fleshliness that characterizes our existence.

A practical and healthy theology of prayer challenges us to envisage our relationship to God in terms of "the body of Christ" or "the temple of God." In this same spirit, Jesus once proclaimed that "I am the vine and you are the branches." God is intimately related to human experience. When we are connected with God, when the "sap" of the vine flows through us, we flourish. When we sever our relationship with God through life-style decisions, destructive values, or faithlessness, then our lives begin to wither.

Prayer points to the immanent activity of a personal God, whose presence in our lives is both creative and responsive. Similar to the mind or spirit, God gives direction and insight to the body of the universe and each of its interrelated members. God addresses us every moment of our lives through insights, inclinations, hunches, images, and challenges. Further, God addresses us indirectly through the events and persons of our lives. As one mystic proclaimed, "all things are the words of God." In the spirit of Jesus' assertion that God is present in the "least of these" (Matthew 25), I would add that all moments are revelatory moments. God has never left Godself without a witness in the world, our minds, or our bodies. Although the divine presence is most often revealed in the unconscious in "sighs too deep for words," times of prayerful reflection enable us to experience consciously certain aspects of God's presence in our lives. The key, however, to experiencing the divine presence and accessing the divine energy is attentiveness to God and the desire to conform as much as possible to God's dynamic will for our lives.

The God who brings life to the body and vitality to the temple works primarily through loving nurture and persuasion. Although the intensity of God's presence may differ from time to time and occasion to occasion according to God's will or the nature of the situation, God always acts in terms of love and not compulsion. The immanent and relational vision of God suggested here is very different from the traditional, hierarchical vision of God that most persons assume is the only possible way to speak about God. According to the traditional vision of God, the primary characteristic of God is God's sovereignty and glory. God's will is the final explanation of everything that occurs in life, be it good fortune and a healthy constitution or cancer or a birth defect. The transcendent God ordains all things and is in complete control. Although God knows everything—past, present, and future, God is unaffected by what goes on in the world. In terms of the metaphor of "the body of Christ," this God can influence the body but it can never feel it! Our prayers ultimately make no difference to God, for nothing that happens in the world truly influences God. Prayer may raise our spirits or enable us to feel closer to our neighbor, but it cannot change anything meaningful in the experience of God. Such prayer enables us only to cope with or accept what God has already willed for us.

In contrast, the vision of God as the animating spirit, immanent in the universe and our lives, sees prayer as an authentic encounter with God. The traditional prayer, "God to whom all hearts are open and all desires known," truly does apply to God. God knows our deepest needs. God feels our pain and rejoices in our success. As the animating spirit of the "body of Christ," God receives and responds to everything that occurs. This incarnational image of God is truly holistic in nature—God relates to the whole and the parts completely, giving and receiving love at every level of existence.

From the perspective of divine intimacy, the traditional doctrines of omnipresence, omniscience, and omnipotence find their true meaning as an inspiration to practical spirituality in this holistic vision of the divine-human relationship. "Omnipresence" means simply that God is right here with us. God is present in the midst of the bread and wine at communion and God is present as the force for healing and reconciliation in every cell of our bodies. "Omniscience," as I've suggested, means that God knows us in such a way that our lives shape God's own experience and creativity in the world.

Prayer becomes most problematic when God is seen either as all powerful or impotent in the world. In either case, prayer is rendered merely a placebo, which may make us and others feel good and, thus, may contribute to our overall health and well-being. Prayer makes no difference to a God who controls everything or is aloof from each thing. The vision of God as the animating spirit of the body of Christ and the one who speaks within our lives in "sighs too deep for words," however, opens us to a multidimensional and relational vision of divine activity. God is powerful, but not all-powerful. God does everything possible to shape our world toward beauty and healing, while yet respecting the freedom and creativity present at every level of existence. God is one of the factors—

indeed, the most significant factor—in the dynamic matrix of events characteristic of each moment's experience as well as the long span of personal and global history. As theologian Marjorie Suchocki asserts, "if God is omnipresent, centering all things, then God is like the rushing water of the universe, filling all spaces, honoring all spaces, centering all spaces, through the specialness of divine presence."[8] The gentle touch of God we experience in prayerful moments permeates the entire universe.

Issues of health and illness as well as the power of prayer are neither one-dimensional nor linear in nature. While God always seeks abundant life in every situation, God is only one of the factors that determines health or illness. As I feel myself coming down with the flu, feeling achy and tired, I am not necessarily a victim of my condition. My ailment is neither entirely my own responsibility nor a reflection of God's attitude toward me. I may take a moment to image God's healing light entering my body with each breath. I may pray for my well-being or ask a friend to lay hands on me or give me a reiki treatment. Depending on how far the flu has progressed, I may only experience a few symptoms or it may disappear entirely. On the other hand, if I am blocked emotionally or spiritually, or let the initial symptoms go too far, I may not be able to access the divine energy that will restore my health. This everyday example reveals the dynamics of prayer and health, which in one way or another present themselves in every prayerful situation, be the focus success at work or the healing of cancer.

The ecology of prayer is profoundly multidimensional. Each prayer is part of a dynamic and relational matrix which minimally includes the following factors: the state of one's physical, emotional, spiritual, and mental health; the impact of the immediate and ambient environment; the influence of the past, both personal and environmental; the nature and progression of the disease; the positive or negative influence of other persons' belief systems; the influence of other persons' prayers and good will as well as one's own spiritual disciplines; the medical treatment utilized; and the presence of God's aim toward abundant life. No one factor is all-determining. When prayers are not answered in terms of our highest ideals, this may be the result of the influence of one or more of the factors on one's immediate situation. Unanswered prayers, accordingly, are not always the result of God's will, but may have their origin in one's own attitudes, one's condition, or the impact of the environment.

Further, it is important to recognize that God is the most significant force in the ecology of prayer. God seeks the good of the whole as well as each constituent part. What appears to be good for one part may be disastrous for neighboring parts. For example, to pray for material abundance may have profound consequences on the ecosystem and the economic well-being of others. We do not own our own prayers, as Marjorie Suchocki notes. They ultimately belong to God and the whole creation.[9] Once we lift our prayers to God, we must trust that God will weave these prayers into the fabric of the universe and the lives of our loved ones in the most creative fashion. As we will see in the next section, one of the goals of a prayerful life is the expansion of self-interest to include others as well as the whole earth and not merely the solitary, individual self.

When our prayers appear to be deferred, the reason may be that it is not yet the right time, either due to the impact of the environment and one's personal history, or God's own sense of our good or the good of the broader community. Just as a parent defers certain wishes of his child, the divine parent seeks those possibilities that are truly best for us and not necessarily those we deem best for ourselves. As Paul notes in Romans, we do not always know what to pray for. We seldom know what is best for ourselves either in the short or long term, and must trust that God is concerned with the totality of our lives. The unanswered prayer may be the prelude to the possibility of a greater good for ourselves and our environment.

An ecological understanding of prayer in "the body of Christ" avoids images of omnipotence and impotence both in terms of God's role in our lives and the impact of our own prayers. Our prayers do make a difference. They open us to God's energetic love as it courses through our lives. In prayer, we gain a wider perspective and a sense of wisdom in terms of our own lives and the well-being of the environment. Acts of power occur when we claim our appropriate place in the "body of Christ" and the divine "vine." The God whose grace speaks in "sighs too deep for words" is enabled to give us new possibilities and greater healing energy when we open ourselves to God. Prayer is an act of partnership in which we respond to God's creative love and commit ourselves to letting that love flow through us in healing energy, insight, wisdom, and loving power.

Prayer opens us to divine energy in all its many forms. But this energy is always contextual and is always influenced by the immediate and long-term environment, which limits, conditions, and supports our highest desires. Divine power is neither omnipotent nor impotent, nor is it the impersonal energy of the new ager or the ambivalent force of the *Star Wars* trilogy. God aims at abundant life personally and globally. In the spirit of the biblical tradition, an ecological image of divine power asserts that God's power influences every heart and every cell, but God's power is also relational and conditioned by the world. Just as our openness to God enables us to do greater things, our openness to God also enables God to do greater things in our lives. The realm of possibilities opens wide when we open to God. In contrast, when we are cut off from God, the divine energy—like the sap in the vine—is prevented from fully expressing itself. In times of spiritual blockage, God does not abandon us, but presents us the best possibilities and greatest energetic support appropriate to the situation. When we are blocked to God's presence, the miracle we seek may not be a mystic vision or a spontaneous healing, but a gradually lifting of the depression or spiritual blockage we feel.

An ecological vision of prayer invites us to partnership with God. When we consciously open ourselves to God in prayer, we support God's will for ourselves and the world and enable God's great love to channel through us.

Prayer as relational cannot be quantified. This is the drawback of those medical studies that attempt to prove the power of prayer. The presence of many pray-ers may open one's life to God in new ways and bring about a healing. Still, prayer operates in an open system and a relational matrix in which even the sustained prayers of a community may fail to yield the hoped for result. Further, God may use even our imperfect and misdirected prayers to bring about an unexpected healing.

Recently, a very popular and highly spiritual member of the university community died of cancer. He was the object of hundreds of prayers and a number of healing services. If anyone should have survived, based on quantitative and even qualitative understandings of the power of prayer, it should have been he. His death was crisis of faith to many of his friends and colleagues, who could not understand *why* he could succumb to cancer. It is important to remember that a multidimensional and relational understanding of prayer does not eliminate the mystery of death and unanswered prayer, but it does place our prayers in a broad perspective and eliminates much of the guilt and anger that accompany unanswered prayer. It also reminds us that God is on our side and that God desires our highest happiness as much as we do.

Finally, in a relational understanding of prayer, God truly hears our deepest prayers. Our joys and sorrows radiate across the entire body of Christ, not only shaping the lives of others but shaping God's own experience. As the philosopher Alfred North Whitehead affirms, God is "the fellow sufferer who understands."[10] God is truly the "abba" who cares for each of us children enough to feel our pain and delight in our joy. We can pray with confidence and live with unanswered prayer precisely because God is praying along with us.

V. The Practice of Prayer and the Power of God

Within the "temple of God," there are many ways to open the doors to God's abundant life. A personal God inspires personal prayers. A global God inspires prayerful attention to the needs of the whole universe. In this section, we will reflect on healthy and life-affirming styles of prayer, which integrate uniqueness and universality in the pray-er's relationship with God and the world. While we may always seek tangible and well-defined answers to prayer, ultimately the goal of prayer is to experience in the upheavals of day-to-day life the words of Mechtild of Magdeburg: "the day of my spiritual awakening was the day I knew all things in God and God in all things."

Although the point of this section is to explore the concrete practice of prayer as a means of promoting spiritual, emotional, physical, and relational health and healing, my remarks will be far from exhaustive. There are many fine books on the practice of prayer which have formed my own spirituality and which promote a holistic vision of the spiritual journey.[11]

At the heart of prayer is the experience of grace. Whether we are aware of it or not, we are connected with God. We are part of the body of Christ: moment by moment and year by year, God is working in our lives. Christ is interceding for us in the womb, on our birth day, and every day of our lives. Even before our first articulated prayer, a still, small voice is praying within us. We do not magically conjure up God as some conjure up spirits or departed loved ones. God is not a genie in bottle who comes at our beck and call. Though God is omnipresent, God is, as C.S. Lewis notes of Aslan, the Christ-figure of the *Chronicles of Narnia*, never "tame." In prayer, we do not seek to control God or even the future, but to discover and follow God's deepest desires within our own deepest desires. Even our invocations in worship are superfluous, if taken literally. God was in the chapel before we arrived. Our invocations are, in fact, our calling out to our own selves to open to God and to pay attention, for we are on holy ground. In fact, our goal is not to pray *to* God but to pray *with* God.

Prayer is not magic; it does not force God's hand. God always desires that we have abundant life. As Jesus proclaims in the Sermon on the Mount, even our moral and religious failings are no impediment to God's care, for God "makes his sun to shine on bad and good people alike" (Matthew 5:45). In contrast to many conservative Christians, this vision of God and prayer strongly maintains that God hears and responds to the prayers of the ardent and the ambivalent, of the orthodox and the heretic, of the faithful and the doubter, of the Christian and the person of another faith tradition. Our prayers of invocation and intercession welcome and invite God to be truly God in our lives and fully God in our world.

When Jesus invites his followers to "ask, seek, and knock" (Matthew 7:7–11), he is calling us to trust that God is already supplying our needs. By opening the doors of our life to God, we are able to receive all that God desires for us, to claim the highest possibilities for health and success, given our current life situation. Prayer is partnership with God. In the divine-human synergy, our prayers enable God's work to be manifest in new and creative ways. Prayer is personal, multidimensional, and relational as it renews our mind and creates within us a new heart. Research on exceptional cancer patients, who survive and flourish despite a terminal prognosis, has noted that exceptional patients are characterized by creativity, flexibility, and receptivity toward others. Prayer is the ultimate exercise in creativity, receptivity, and flexibility. In the spirit of the biblical tradition, those who take prayer seriously must be willing to transform their lives in accordance with the divine-human adventure to which they are committed. Adventurous prayer calls us to go beyond our needs and our limited view of the self in order to claim the whole universe as relevant to our well-being. In such prayer, the self is not lost. Rather, the narrow self dies so that a cosmic and deathless vision of self, committed to the well-being of all, is born. Prayer is an exercise of connectedness by which we affirm our place in the body of Christ and the divinely rooted vine.

The best advice that can be given to anyone seeking a creative and health-affirming prayer life comes from the British Benedictine Dom Chapman, "pray as you can, not as you can't." A personal God creates each one of us personally and uniquely. While certain prayer forms have brought healing and spiritual growth through the ages, no one form is final. Prayer is a process and, as the Zen proverb suggests, we must not confuse "the moon with the finger pointing toward it." As a dynamic process, our prayer lives combine ritual and novelty, tradition and uniqueness, habit and spontaneity.

For many persons, the greatest impediment to healthy prayer is perfectionism. Many of us feel like spiritual babies, fearful of revealing our inexperience or difficulties to God or another person. Yet, the heart of prayer is simply "simplicity." Meister Eckhart asserted that if the only prayer you can make is "thank you," this will be enough. For one who is drowning or escaping a burning house, long and complicated prayers or subtle meditative techniques are useless—crying "help" is enough! The prayer of simplicity involves bringing our lives just as we are to God. The Psalms are wonderful tools for prayer. Nothing is excluded or edited out—anger, depression, fear, hatred, celebration, joy are all brought before God. As selfish as it may seem, simple petitions ("I need this, God") may serve over the long run to purify one's heart and one's desire.

Our needs are important to God. By praying our needs for health, good relationships, financial success, job security, we discover the true and deep desires of our hearts. As we begin to pray our needs, we should hold nothing back from God, however small or however large. The one whose "eye is on the sparrow" is surely watching over us. Yet, even as we focus on our own needs, we are called to take a moment to ask simply "God, show me what is important...God, show me what I really need." Such focus, even if it is only on our needs, brings God into our life and allows the divine energy to transform our needs and our focus to include others and the good of the whole. Often, we do not know what we truly need or what is best for ourselves in the immediate moment or in the long run. Simply opening to God gives us an expanded awareness of the relationship of the present to the future and the possibilities and pitfalls of certain courses of action.

As we explore the concept of prayer within the global body of Christ, we realize that we are connected with every member of the body. As the apostle Paul proclaims, "if one part of the body suffers, all the other parts of the body suffer with it; if one part of the body is praised, all the other parts share its happiness" (1 Corinthians 12:26). Intercession is an essential companion to petition in an expanding and health-giving practice of prayer. Our prayers for others radiate across the universe. They not only surround the other in the healing light of God, as Randolph Byrd's studies on the power of prayer indicate, they also create an openness that enables God to be more active in the healing process.

There is no one technique of intercessory prayer that fits all persons and situations. We may simply cry out for help for another person without expecting a particular outcome. We may also pray for healing, success, or prosperity, while leaving the outcome in the hands of God and the healing environment. On the other hand, we may use our imagination to envisage a particular outcome. Agnes Sanford, one of the pioneers in the restoration of the healing ministry in mainstream Christianity, reminds us to image those we pray for as healthy and whole. When I pray for someone's recovery or for the successful outcome to one of her or his projects, I often simply see them as surrounded by the light of God and ask God to give them the grace and healing they need in that time and place.

Both intercession and petition are acts of hope, grounded in the belief that the future is open and a new creation lies on the horizon. Hopelessness has been connected with the breakdown of the immune system. In contrast, hope is "the moral equivalent of war" (to quote William James) for those who suffer. It enlivens, empowers, and encourages persons to help shape the future and to be cocreators in the incarnation of God's will in one's life and in the world. As theologian Walter Wink asserts, "history belongs to the intercessors....The future belongs to whoever can envision in the manifold of its potentials a new and desirable possibility, which faith then fixes on as inevitable....Hope envisages its future and then acts as if that future is now irresistible, thus helping to create the reality for which it longs."[12]

Imagination is an important element in hope-giving prayer. Old Testament scholar Walter Bruggemann speaks of the "prophetic imagination" as a countercultural movement within biblical spirituality. Prayer is always countercultural in nature. In times of crisis or complacency, prayer envisages an alternative future. Within the circles of Religious Science, Unity, and the new age movement, persons are counseled to envisage themselves as already experiencing a desirable future. The prayerful imagination involves seeing oneself or another as healthy and robust, as succeeding at a job interview, as resolving a particular problem. Often before I preach or enter the classroom to lecture, I imagine myself speaking words of wisdom and insight and visualize the students and congregation being blessed and educated by my words. As I drive across campus for the Sunday Chapel Services at Georgetown, I imagine the students awakening and rejoicing in the day, and ask that God lead those persons who most need to hear the message and share in the sacraments to be directed to church that morning. As a friend takes an exam or interviews for a job, I can imagine my friend surrounded by the light of God. Nearly every night, I take a moment as I look in on my sleeping son to visualize God surrounding him with light, love, and inspiration.

Imagination is at the heart of many cancer recovery programs. If imagination can enhance healing during times of crisis, it can be just as effective in health maintenance and prevention of illness. Visualize yourself as healthy, compassionate, vital, wise, and intelligent. See the divine light permeating every organ and cell. Imagine yourself eating healthy foods. Imagination is a tool by which we recognize God's presence in our lives. For example, one can image Jesus as one's companion, walking beside and providing constant guidance and protection. In times of weakness and pain, one can visualize God carrying oneself amid the crisis. In such moments, the words of the poem "Footprints" become a lived reality.

No moment of life is immune from prayer. One can, with Brother Lawrence, encounter God in the ordinary moments of cooking and cleaning. Many persons take time as they cook to image and pray for each person who will dine at their table. Others take a moment for prayer as they answer the phone or meet a friend. As I walk across campus, I often silently bless the people I meet with words I've learned from Maxie

Dunnam, "I give Christ to and receive Christ from you."

Our anguish is also meant to be taken to God. Painful moments call us to prayer. The Psalmist (Psalm 22:1) and Jesus (Mark 15:34) cry out "my God, my God, why hast Thou forsaken me?" Such prayers do not always diminish the pain. They are not meant to be means of escape or denial. Rather, they open our hearts to God's merciful presence amid the pain. Although God is not the cause of our personal sorrow, God both experiences and acts within our most desperate situations. As we pray our pain, we may discover God's own prayer within our pain. Further, our pain itself can become, like the cross of Jesus, our own offering to God. Authentic spirituality does not deliver us from evil, it transforms the evils we face by placing them in the divine context and opening them to the flow of divine love. As we discover God within our suffering, we find new hope and we experience an expansion of ourselves in which our pain becomes joined with God's pain and the pain of the world. Further, since pain typically constricts our attention span, the spaciousness of spirit that results from prayerful living may, in fact, reduce the physical pain we feel.

Contrary to some new age thinking which identifies spiritual growth with harmony and peace alone, prayer, at times, may bring greater pain and discomfort into our lives. The deepest mental and spiritual healing may require the deepest pain for its transformation. Openhearted prayer awakens us to the cries of the poor and the needs of our neighbor. Openhearted prayer connects us with both joy and sorrow. The sorrows of the world, viewed from our window, the TV, the inner city, the front page, are no longer foreign. They are our pain as well, for the pain of the world is the body of Christ. Yet, the tragedies of life do not overwhelm or victimize us, for in our praying, we discover that we can make a difference and that there are resources for transformation within ourselves and within the constantly open system of the body of Christ. As we pray in partnership with God, we may discover that our role in the body of Christ is similar to certain cells in our body's circulatory and immune systems—to answer the prayers of others by confronting evils, bringing nourishment, and providing protection.

The final prayer form I want to suggest is simply the prayer of open receptivity. All prayer makes a difference. However, some studies suggest that the most effective prayers are those that simply say "thy will be done" or place oneself complete-ly within the divine purpose. Such prayers of open receptivity are far from passive or fatalistic. To pray for the realization of God's will is to ask that one be attentive to God's deepest desire in a particular context and that one's thoughts, prayers, and actions follow and support God's desire. Prayers of open receptivity seek to embody what the theologian Paul Tillich called "theonomous" spirituality. We desire to be one with God in our intent. We also desire that the world reflect the will of God. Such prayers do not abrogate our freedom or respon-sibility. They may even call us to adventure and transforma-tion, since God is always doing a new thing. Within the matrix of the moment in all of its many dimensions, we wish to be attentive to God's voice. In listening for the one voice amid the many voices, we discover a "way where there is no way" and find ourselves on holy ground right where we are standing.

"Thy will be done" prayers may be the most effective sim-ply because they aim to align themselves fully with God's will. If God knows us better than we know ourselves and if God seeks the highest possibilities for us and the events of the world, given the current state of reality as well as the uncer-tain future, then focusing simply on listening and following creates an open space where the divine incarnation can be realized, and where an event can become truly an act of God and humankind.

As we align ourselves with God, even the unanswered prayer can become a means of spiritual growth and a revelation of grace. The apostle Paul speaks of a "thorn in the flesh" that is not relieved regardless of how often or diligently he prays. Even mystical experiences cannot deliver him from his anguish. However, in the midst of his struggle he receives a word from God. He recognizes his own dependence on God and, I believe, interdependence with the larger body of Christ and proclaims in God's voice, "my grace is sufficient for you and my power is made perfect in your weakness" (2 Corinthians 12:9). Prayer will not deliver us from death or insure success in all our endeavors, but it will open us to a horizon in which God's grace moves creatively in every encounter and our lives become part of God's cosmic embodiment. In that prayerful encounter, the temple of God is cleansed and made whole even in the midst of suffering.

QUESTIONS FOR REFLECTION AND DISCUSSION

1) What is your response to the recent studies on the power of prayer? Do you think that prayer really makes a difference in the physical and spiritual lives of persons?

2) How do you respond to the advice that physicians should pray for their patients? Do you think that such prayers might compromise their medical objectivity?

3) Does God answer the prayers of non-Christians?

4) What prayer forms have been most helpful in your own spiritual journey? What forms have been least helpful?

5) How do you understand unanswered prayer?

6) What is your response to the idea that God is not all-powerful and that God may need our prayers to be more effective in certain situations?

7) Do our prayers really influence God? Can we, conversely, experience God's influence in our own lives?

CHAPTER FIVE

IN SEARCH
OF THE MIRACULOUS

I. Signs and Wonders?

When I was a young boy, growing up in California's Salinas Valley, my favorite solitary pastime was throwing a rubber ball against the side of our house while I dreamed of being a major league pitcher or a professional quarterback. More often than not, I would eventually lose the ball in the flowers and bushes that surrounded our home. If I couldn't find the ball, I often called upon God in prayers and challenges. "God, help me find my baseball." When I became especially frustrated, I would cry out in despair, "God, if you exist, let me find it!" My childish faith was sorely tried when neither prayer nor searching could yield the lost ball. I had expected divine intervention, a miracle on my behalf, and I couldn't imagine why it did not occur.

We are an age that expects miracles. Although many of us have abandoned the healings of the biblical world as superstitious vestiges of a bygone era, we still expect divine and technological interventions that will restore our health and solve all of our problems. The discipline necessary for good health is often too demanding. The patience that prayer requires involves too much faith and delayed gratification. Whether the source be God, the physician, or the latest technological breakthrough, many of us expect instant results and instant answers to life's deepest issues. When the answers don't come or the healing does not occur, we often become disillusioned and lose faith in God, medicine, or the goodness of the universe.

Disillusionment and the shattering of our expectations are always painful. However, the religious path has always recognized the importance of disillusionment as the first step toward authentic faith and the experience of God's blessings. When we are dis-illusioned, that is, free of our illusions, we begin to see life as it is and God as God is. Then we will more fully understand the nature of the miraculous and our role in asking for and receiving miracles. While we may depend on miracles for our salvation, we will no longer expect them on our terms and timetable.

It is appropriate to conclude this book with a theological reflection on the miraculous. Miracles are the business of religion, scoffer and believer proclaim from their respective standpoints. As I remember my own childhood, there was an aura of the miraculous surrounding prayer and worship at our home. "I believe in miracles," purred the television evangelist Kathryn Kuhlman. "Expect a miracle," shouted the faith healer Oral Roberts. "Put your hand on the television set as a point of contact while I pray," invited another television healer. In the piety of my childhood, I dreamed of the miraculous intervention of a miracle-working God. Though my brother and I often made fun of the antics of the television healers, we still expected divine interventions that would enable us to find a lost baseball or escape the wrath of the local bullies or help our team win the game in the final inning. While today I realize that my childhood petitions for divine intervention were no doubt simplistic and immature, I recognize there is still a child in each of us that waits for a miracle of deliverance or an unexpected solution to life's problems.

Singer-songwriter Paul Simon notes that we live in "the age of miracle and wonder." What our grandparents could only imagine has become a reality for us—x-rays, cellular phones, fax machines, bypass surgery, and organ transplantation. Humans travel into outer space and chart the geography of the galaxies. The impossible and the incredible for earlier generations have become the everyday, and we wonder what new miracles will burst forth in our lifetimes or the lifetimes of our children.

Where once God alone could produce a miracle, understood as a decisive act of power and grace for our salvation and well-being, humankind now speaks of its own miraculous powers as we predict the future, alter the boundaries of life and death, change weather patterns, and fathom the mysteries of black holes and quantum particles. "Acts of God" have been replaced by acts of human technological creativity and "the hand of God" has been reduced to the nimble fingers of the surgeon. In many ways, we have become the miracle workers as the realms of mystery and unilateral divine activity recede before our own ambitious powers and insight.

Still, in times of crisis and uncertainty, our personal and technological sense of self-sufficiency and omnipotence disappears. The need for a miracle from beyond ourselves becomes paramount. We pray for a sign or wonder, whether it comes from the hand of God or a technological breakthrough employed by the physician in the operating room. In such moments, we feel both hopeful and vulnerable, because in our pain and disillusionment we realize, perhaps for the first time, that we cannot make it on our own. We need help from a higher power—be it God, a guru or charismatic leader, an energetic cosmic force, or a concerned and competent professional.

To the religious person, the boundaries of life and our own powers are invitations to petitionary and intercessory prayer. Prayer is always in search of miracles, whether those miracles involve transformation of the present moment, relief of pain, deliverance from addiction, or a greater experience of God's presence and power in our lives.

Historically, the quest for the miraculous has centered around religious and medical practices. If we go back to the dawn of human history or visit the ancient habitats of native or aboriginal peoples, we discover the essential unity of religion and medicine. The earliest healers, such as the shaman, became wounded healers through their confrontation and transformation of death and disease. Dwelling in an enchanted and lively universe, the shaman and medicine person experienced disease as a meaningful revelation of the spiritual life of the person and her or his tribal unit. In bringing the heavenly harmony back to earth, the shaman reunited her or his patient with the healing balm of the universe. This same shamanic ritual is still implicitly or explicitly reenacted in every healing ritual, whether it be a bedside prayer, a quiet service of healing and communion, a revival meeting, or a medical intervention.

While few physicians are priests today, physicians still command our awe because of their power over life and death. We are intrigued by the physician's art and call upon the M.D. as if his or her title really meant "medical deity" when illness threatens our well-being or survival. Nearly every Thursday evening, millions of Americans are mesmerized by the frenetic and fast-paced television drama, *E.R.* Each program reveals the miracles of medical technology. Patients are literally brought back from the dead by the employment of heart paddles and medication.

While we marvel at the commitment and ability of the medical team, there is a dark side to *E.R.* and the world of medical wonders that lies just beneath its apparently miraculous surface. The physicians portrayed are often troubled and ambivalent about their own powers. The death of a patient is an occasion for confusion and guilt. Even if death is inevitable, its occurrence challenges the competence of the physician and the philosophical worldview of western medicine itself. Surrounded by the technological wonders of the emergency room, the medical staff often forgets that eventually every one of its patients will die. Though we may eradicate particular illnesses, we can never eradicate death itself.

A similar dynamic is at work in the many television programs highlighting Christian faith healers and divine miracle working. Yet, this time it is the patient who is left to feel guilty. In one form or another, those who are left unhealed hear the constant refrain, "if only you'd trusted God, you would have been healed....if only you were generous in your gifts to the healer's ministry, your child would have survived....if only you had more faith, you would be well....if only...."

While subscribing to a radically different worldview from the evangelical faith healer, new age healers often suggest the same dynamic of health and illness. Persons at their most vulnerable hear new age litanies such as: "You create your own reality....If you're sick, it must be your fault....Think positively, use your affirmations, and you will be healed....You are 100% responsible for your life." When the healing does not occur, guilt, cynicism, and disillusionment undermine what little hope a person has left. Worse, I am a failure in my own quest for healing, and not even God or my higher self will help me!

Today, despite the quest for miraculous cures, there is much cynicism about healing. The televangelists often seem to be little more than telemarketers in search of the resources of those gullible enough to buy their products. Many new age healers make unrealistic promises and use the term "healer" so indiscriminately that the word has lost its meaning and credibility. Physicians, despite their technological success, often seem to be detached and uncaring, merely technicians during life's most critical moments. Health crises challenge their own status as healers.

Still, we seek the miraculous. We yearn for deliverance from our ills. We hunger for something or someone to believe in when all else has failed us. We want to experience a sign or wonder, an act of power, that will bring us relief and the hope of new life. Like the young boy searching for his lost ball, we cry out, "God, if you exist, please save me, please heal me!"

Today, there is a great need for a credible theology of miracles and healing that will encourage faith and support our physical and spiritual well-being, and yet avoid unrealistic expectations. Sound theological reflection will deliver us from the linear approach to healing that encourages easy answers and magical thinking. It also opens us to the multidimensional realm of divine-human relatedness, where we can depend on a miracle—but never demand one!

Today, more than a few physicians—Bernie Siegel, Deepak Chopra, Dale Matthews—are sounding like preachers as they go in quest of a new kind of miracle, an act of power grounded in the integration of science and faith. Bernie Siegel speaks of "love, medicine, and miracles" and proclaims that "all healing is related to the ability to give and accept unconditional love."[1] Siegel believes that when persons integrate love, spiritual exploration, and medicine, miracles happen—spontaneous remissions occur, relationships are healed, prognoses are updated and extended, and persons die with joy and faith.

At the heart of this book is the belief that medicine and religion can no longer live in separate worlds. They must once more be reunited, as they were in the ancient world, in the common quest for healing. Persons of faith are challenged theologically and personally to explore the impact of the body on spiritual well-being. Physicians and scientists are challenged to recognize the significance of faith, prayer, community, and values in the health of persons and communities. A truly holistic approach to health includes prayer and prozac, meditation and medication, affirmations and antibiotics. While persons will be encouraged to prepare themselves for the miraculous, they will also understand that miracles come in many forms— some dramatic, some spiritual, and some gradual. Indeed, the greatest miracle may be the gift of seeing God's presence in all things, even when sickness and death strike the temple of God.

II. The Miraculous Christ

Until the nineteenth century, most Christians believed that miracles were at the heart of Jesus' ministry. Jesus healed the leper, gave sight to the blind, and raised the dead. According to the traditional understanding of Christian faith, Jesus' miracles, including the resurrection, authenticated his claim to be the Messiah, God's Chosen One, and manifested his uniqueness as God's son. But, with the rise of modern science and materialistic thinking, Jesus' healing ministry has become an embarrassment to many Christians. On the one hand, many Christians are appalled by the vision of a God who acts arbitrarily and unilaterally to heal his apparent favorites. They can no longer affirm the viewpoint that miracles are divine interventions, given by divine fiat to the favored few, in an otherwise mechanistic universe. Further, many Christians see the hope for miraculous interventions as discouraging human responsibility. When we superstitiously hope that God will save us from our problems, we turn our backs on a world that needs our commitment. Still other Christians affirm the dualism of mind and body and hold that the only proper work of the church is the salvation of souls, the counseling of the troubled, or social welfare projects.

The modern worldview and its focus on observable and linear causes has left virtually no room for the power of prayer or healing acts. Many modern biblical scholars, such as Rudolf Bultmann and John Dominic Crossan, influenced by this mechanistic and linear understanding of reality, have seen the miracles of Jesus either as vestiges of the superstitious supernaturalism of the earliest Christians or metaphors for the healing of the spirit and social order. Jesus' true healing message, they claim, involved the transformation of the social order, the acceptance of the outcast, and the invitation to experience authentically the presence of God. If prayer and laying on of hands make any difference at all, they assert, it is solely at the level of the mind and spirit and not physical existence. Such theologians and their followers insist that Jesus' interest in health is an invitation for Christians today to seek just social structures and universal health care, but not the dramatic healing of the sick. This is a scientific matter to be carried out by physicians, and ultimately not an issue of faith or spiritual discipline.

It is clear from the perspective of this book that such one-dimensional and dualistic images of Jesus' ministry are no longer justified. They themselves are a vestige of the mechanistic and materialistic worldview that has been superseded by the multidimensional world of quantum physics and ecological thinking. The vision of the universe as the dynamic, relational, and multidimensional body of Christ suggested in this book leaves room for the power of prayer, the integration of spirituality and physical well-being, and the surprising acts of healing power traditionally known as miracles. Jesus' ministry of healing at every level of life is, in fact, the primary manifestation of God's presence in the body of Christ corporately and each temple of God personally.

The most casual reader of the gospels will soon discover that the earliest Christians understood Jesus as a healer and miracle worker. Miracles abounded wherever Jesus went. These miracles encompassed the whole of human life. They transformed minds as well as bodies and healed spirits as well as social and political relations. Jesus' ministry was truly holistic: it called for saved persons, with saved spirits and bodies, living in a saved society. The hallmark of Jesus' ministry is found in Luke's account of Jesus' first sermon: "the Spirit of the Lord is upon me...to preach good news to the poor...to proclaim release to the captives and recovery of sight to the blind and to set at liberty those who are oppressed" (Luke 4:18).

According to biblical scholars, nearly one-fifth of the gospel accounts of Jesus' ministry relate to healing of mind, body, and spirit. In contrast to Hebraic theology of his day and many Christian and new age philosophies of our own time, that see health as the result of righteousness or spiritual advancement and disease as the result of sin or ignorance, Jesus saw health and illness as multidimensional in nature. The God who promised abundant life did not punish people with illness, but sought their salvation and healing. In describing Jesus' healing ministry, Francis MacNutt, one of the pioneers of the healing revival in the Roman Catholic Church, proclaims that "never do we find that Jesus, in the presence of sickness, encourages people to accept their sickness, nor did Jesus give them sermonettes on patience and endurance. Instead, His example was that every time he met with sickness, he treated it as an evil."[2] The good news of God's coming reign was embodied in Jesus' healing of the whole person in this life as well as the next.

In contrast to many of today's healers, who often focus on just one method of accessing the miraculous, Jesus utilized no one particular healing technique. Jesus transformed broken persons through touch, words of forgiveness, exorcisms of demons (some of which might today be described in terms of multiple personality disorders or schizophrenia), verbal commands, anointing, and the faith of those who encountered him. For Jesus, every moment was miraculous and every encounter was an epiphany of the healing God. God can use any medium to bring about healing, since, as Jesuit poet Gerard Manley Hopkins proclaims, "the world is charged with the grandeur of God." While we cannot fully discern the mechanics of Jesus' healing power, we can assume that extraordinary divine energy was at his disposal and could be channeled toward persons in spiritual, emotional, or physical distress. Jesus' healing energy is the revelation in its most decisive manifestation of the omnipresent energy of God's love.

Jesus' own promise to his disciples challenges those Christians who believe that the age of healing ended with the first century. Jesus' followers are called to reveal God's healing power in their time and place, even in this technological age. "Whoever believes in me will also do the works that I do; and greater than these will he do, because I go to the Father" (John 14:12–13). The universality of Christ's healing ministry is noted by Francis MacNutt, who asserts that Jesus' assumption was that "extraordinary actions will be performed by ordinary persons."[3] Yet, Jesus was a healer and not a magician. Magic seeks to bend the divine will and the universe to our particular needs, while authentic healing is grounded in a personal encounter with a personal God and an alignment with God's purpose.

Today, the spiritual and scientific geography of the universe is being transformed. Relationship, novelty, and creativity have replaced isolation, materialism, and mechanism as the primary metaphors for understanding the universe. The vision of the universe as the body of Christ, animated by the indwelling spirit of God, affirms the essential relatedness of body and spirit and makes room for the presence and activity of God in every event. While we no longer need to wait passively for supernatural interventions from the outside to deliver us from our troubles, we can still confidently seek the guidance and healing presence of the God who is embodied in each moment of existence.

Jesus' ministry challenges persons to be in partnership with God as cocreators of miraculous and health-giving events. Such miracles are not violations of the laws of nature, but surprising and transformative revelations of the God whose grace is ever-present within the universe. The miraculous arises not from an external and sporadic supernatural intervention, but from a heightening of God's presence within the constellation of events, including a person's openness to the divine, the environment, the prayers of others, and our own personal condition. While all moments reveal the miracle of God's presence, some moments more fully reveal the depths of God's love for creation. These are the moments in history and in our own lives we describe as unique, powerful, and miraculous. In these moments, bodies are healed, sins forgiven, and spirits renewed.

III. Creating Miracles

Today, the interest in the miraculous is found among the educated and affluent as well as the uneducated and impoverished. Venturing beyond the wonders of technology, persons seek the guidance of angels, study near death experiences, and expect miracles in times of personal crisis. Recently, two authors—Dan Wakefield and Carolyn Miller—have spoken of the possibility of "creating miracles." While I do not believe that persons can "create" miracles on their own, I do believe that we can participate as cocreators with God by aligning ourselves with God's graceful movements in our lives.

Dan Wakefield believes that we can create an atmosphere in which the miracles of transformation and healing are more likely to occur by awakening ourselves to the miracles of everyday existence.[4] Wakefield sees the extraordinary acts of transformation as a revelation of reality at its deepest level. Wakefield affirms the spirit of Einstein, who states that "there are only two ways to live your life. One is as though nothing is a miracle. The other is as if everything is a miracle."[5] When persons wake up to the holiness and guidance present in all things, miracles happen.

Carolyn Miller believes that if miracles are real, then learning to access them is crucial. The occurrence of miracles is related to the shift of our experience to a peaceful, expansive, and open state of consciousness. "By entering a peaceful, meditative state of consciousness, we make it possible for God to guide us into changing our physical reality."[6] Miller suggests that there is a "miracle-prone personality," characterized by trust, strength, imagination, optimism, and the ability to shift to a peaceful state of consciousness. Miracles happen more often to persons who live in a manner congruent with their inner selves.[7] According to Miller, "miracles are the result of a collaboration between our creative ability and divine guidance."[8] In the spirit of the previous chapter, I believe that miracles occur when we align ourselves prayerfully with the will of God and discover our place in the dynamic body of Christ.

Francis MacNutt points out that extraordinary things happen when ordinary persons open themselves to God. Indeed, because of our blindness and self-absorption, we may miss out on the majority of divine moments in our lives. The miracles in my own life have been, for the most part, undramatic, yet quite meaningful. Still, one physical transformation stands out. For a number of years, every several months I would have a debilitating headache, followed by an attack of nausea. After suffering these infrequent, yet painful, episodes for many years, I decided to do something about it. I realized that I did not need to be a victim of this condition and that, by God's grace and my own spiritual efforts, I would find relief. As the headache and nausea emerged, I chose to spend the day in the centering prayer, described earlier in this book. With every breath, I intoned, "I breathe the spirit deeply in and blow it peacefully out again." Though I experienced waves of nausea, I responded to them with a breath prayer, until finally they subsided. These attacks have never returned. Later, in the course of another time of meditation, I discovered that the source of the illness was a childhood experience of car sickness. In the language of the faith healers, a miracle of healing had occurred—a physical ailment as well as an unconscious, yet powerful, memory was healed.

Much more dramatic is the story of a woman diagnosed with an advanced and almost always fatal case of cancer. Rather than waiting for death or disability, she turned to God, her friends in church, and to her own spiritual resources. Through an integration of visualization exercises in which she focused on the healing light of God permeating every cell of her body, meditative and petitionary prayer, exercise, and diet, along with the prayers of her church and the laying on of hands by Christian healers, she experienced a remission. Although she also utilized medication and regularly consulted with her physician, she attributes her healing to the love of God and the openness of her friends and herself to divine healing.

Many persons have found healing through the liturgical acts of the church—the laying on of hands and the eucharist. Although God is present everywhere as the power of love and healing, certain acts and places are charged with divine power. While we cannot explain the reason these ritual acts and holy places are set apart, it is my belief that their uniqueness arises from the interplay of God's own choice to be more dynamically present in certain venues as well as the spiritual field of force created by the historical openness of persons to look for God's presence when they receive a healing touch or the eucharist.

One such place of divine healing is Lourdes. According to tradition, the Virgin Mary appeared there to a young French girl, Bernadette Soubirous, and told her of her desire to have a chapel erected in the grotto at Lourdes. Over the years, millions have come to the springs at Lourdes seeking healing and recovery from chronic and terminal illnesses. Although the waters contain no curative properties from a medical point of view, thousands have received healing as a result of their pilgrimage to Lourdes. Still, fewer than one hundred of these healings have been declared as miracles, according to the strict standards of the medical commission at Lourdes.

In order for a healing to be considered a miracle, the following conditions must have existed: 1) the malady must be a grave one, 2) the malady must not have been in decline, 3) no medication was utilized or the medication was ineffectual, 4) the cure was sudden and instantaneous, 5) the cure was complete, 6) the cure could not have come from a natural cause, 7) there was no relapse following the cure.[9] According to Ruth Cranston, a Protestant chronicler of the healings at Lourdes, "the miracle is characterized by an extreme acceleration of the processes of organic repair."[10]

Although the miracles at Lourdes are attributed to divine intervention, even these miracles involve a person's openness to God. According to Cranston, persons are often cured when they let go and surrender completely to God. Similar to the idea of "creating miracles," persons at Lourdes "receive miracles," when they: 1) no longer think of themselves and their cure, 2) focus their prayers on others, and 3) give themselves up to God altogether.[11]

The images of "miracle-prone personalities," of liturgical healing, and healing places such as Lourdes invite persons to create and receive their own miracles. (Among new agers, Sedona, Arizona; Glastonbury, England; and Iona and Findhorn, Scotland, have been invested with healing powers.)

Though there is no one path to the experience of these acts of divine power, persons may open themselves to divine energy by immersing themselves in prayer and supplication, by awakening to a larger perspective on life, and by utilizing the prayers of the faithful. This is *not* the result of magic or human effort, but the experience of a power beyond ourselves gracefully and unexpectedly entering our lives. In many ways, every miracle can be understood as an answer to prayer in terms of the dynamics discussed in chapter four.

The biblical tradition gives us three approaches to the creation of miracles. If all of reality is miraculous at its depths, as the reflection of divine wisdom and creativity, then the first step to experiencing a decisive act of healing is recognizing that any situation and venue can be a catalyst for healing. The story is told of Naaman, the commander of the Syrian army. Suffering from leprosy, he sought out the Hebrew judge, Elisha. Naaman, however, became angry when the prophet advised him to wash in the Jordan River seven times, rather than a more impressive river or healing spot. Eventually Naaman is transformed when he listens to the words of his servants: "if the prophet had commanded you to do some great thing, would not you have done it? How much rather, then, when he says to you, 'Wash and be clean'?" (2 Kings 5:13). As soon as Naaman dipped himself in the waters, he became healthy once more. The processes of healing may not be complicated. If God has placed a bias toward health and well-being at the heart of reality, then the movements of healing are omnipresent and omniactive. Accordingly, physical health, spiritual healing, and miraculous experiences often result from simply following the directions—be it in the area of diet, spiritual guidance, or prayer. But, even though our openness to God makes a difference, the healing, be it dramatic or long-term, comes in God's way and on God's terms and not merely our own.

Persons often receive miraculous healings when they finally realize that they have no other options but to seek God's
grace. When Jesus addresses the man who waited thirty-eight
years for a healing at the Pool of Bethesda, he asks him "Do
you want to be healed?" (John 5:6). When the man gives his
excuses for the failure of healing, Jesus simply tells him to do
the impossible, "Stand up, take your bed, and walk." Healing
may be costly. It may mean letting go of being a victim and
claiming one's own responsibility for life. It may mean no
longer making excuses for one's situation and taking action to
change one's life. To many persons, the familiar habits and illnesses that block God's healing love are often more comfortable than the call to adventure, transformation, and insecurity
that healing requires. But our excuses collapse when we
answer "yes," with all our doubts, to the simple question, "do
you want to be healed? do you *really* want to be healed?"

Miracles and acts of power occur when human faith
encounters the power of God. The synoptic gospels tell of a
woman with chronic hemorrhage (Matthew 9:20–22, Mark
5:25–34, Luke 8:43–46). Like many then and now, she received
no relief from medical care. She was nearly bankrupt from the
medical bills. Yet, when she saw Jesus, she took one more
chance: "If I touch even the hem of his garment, I shall be
made well" (Mark 5:28). As she touched Jesus, she experienced an immediate healing. Jesus, in turn, felt her presence in
terms of a power that had gone out from him. As the manifestation of divine love and wisdom, Jesus is a dynamic and
empowering energy source for those in need of healing.
Through her faith, the woman opens to the divine energy that
will heal her. Jesus responds with the words, "Daughter, your
faith has made you well; go in peace, and be healed of your
disease" (Mark 5:34). She "created" her miracle by trusting
God and risking disappointment one more time. While there
are no guarantees that healing will occur as we expect, healing

energy is released as a result of desiring healing, trusting God, and accepting healing on God's terms and not our own.

The creation of miracles is not merely the result of a solitary commitment or an individual relationship with God. Whether in the hospital or the chapel, miracles arise from the healing commitment of a community. Just as there are miracle-prone persons, there are also miracle-prone communities. Miracle-prone communities are high touch as well as high tech. They are communities whose members are committed to nurturing the spiritual resources of each member through prayer, dialogue, and participation in the healing arts.

Our cries for deliverance are heard and may even transform God's own perspective of our situation or the situation of another. The Gospels note a strange and, at first glance, unflattering encounter between Jesus and a Canaanite woman (Matthew 15:21–28; Mark 7:24–30). When she begs Jesus to heal her demon-possessed daughter, Jesus initially rejects her plea with harsh words, "I was sent only to the lost sheep of the house of Israel....It is not fair to take the children's bread and throw it to the dogs." But, after she protests that "even the dogs eat the crumbs that fall from the master's table," Jesus himself is amazed by her faith and heals her daughter. While it may be difficult to believe, our prayers may, in fact, change God's intention for a particular situation. The challenge to "ask, seek, and knock" reveals the dynamic divine-human partnership in which both partners are constantly transforming one another. This is not magic, but a lively and loving relationship in which our prayers open up new possibilities for God's healing work in our world.

IV. Healing and Curing

Today, persons are discovering that healing and curing are not necessarily the same thing. Curing—either by prayer or medical intervention—pertains only to the physical body, whereas healing involves the well-being of the entire person, with special emphasis on her or his spiritual well-being. Indeed, it is possible to be healed spiritually even when one is not cured physically. This is the goal of spiritually based hospices for the terminally ill. Miracle-prone communities create an environment in which healing can occur at the levels where it is needed most. Within the body of Christ, God's presence is more fully felt and more effectual wherever persons are emotionally, physically, and spiritually nurtured. A truly miracle-prone community becomes a mini-Lourdes or eucharistic community as it breaks down the obstacles to experiencing God's love.

Studies have indicated that members of religious communities live healthier and longer lives. Further, it has been found that women with cancer have a higher rate of remission and survival when they are active members of support groups. The spirituality of the group opens and supports one's own spiritual life. This not only enhances the immune system but creates an open space in which God can be more effectively present.

The notion of a healing or miracle-prone community has significant implications for the care of the hospitalized. While good hospital care is grounded in advanced technology, it is completed by spiritual nurture, caring professionals, and the prayers and visitations of loving friends. Everything possible must be done to create a physical as well as spiritual environment, from favorite pictures to music and videotapes, to pastoral visitations by friends and clergy, to training in meditation and visualization. In its integration of advanced technology and the healing touch, the hospital of the future will resemble the ancient Greek Asclepian temples where people received both spiritual and physical healing. Persons of faith as well as physicians will affirm that God is the source of all healing, whether it is stimulated by prayer, the laying on of hands, chemotherapy, or surgery.

IV. When the Miracle Doesn't Come

C.S. Lewis notes that Lazarus was, in fact, a tragic as well as fortunate person—he received new life, yet he had to die twice! While we can affirm that all things are permeated by the miraculous power of God, often the miracles we seek do not occur. Chronic illness, depression, cancer, and AIDS persist, despite our prayers and supplications and the support of a healing community.

I know the challenge of unanswered prayer and the failure of a miracle from personal experience. In 1990, my mother, aged 71, went into surgery to mend a broken hip. Throughout the day of her surgery, from three thousand miles away, I lifted her up in prayer and asked God's blessings upon her and my father. I trusted that she would be well and expected to speak with her soon, until I heard the unexpected and heartbreaking words, "A blood clot broke loose and your mother has died." There were no answers, only the agonized prayers of the Psalmist, "where were you God? why have you forsaken me and my family?" However, at her funeral, I received an insight that even in death, my mother was in God's hands as the congregation sang the words of the old hymn, "It Is Well With My Soul":

"When peace, like a river, attendeth my way,
when sorrows, like sea billows roll;
whatever my lot, thou hast taught me to say,
It is well, it is well, with my soul."

This was the faith she lived by and the faith she died by. Although I grieved my loss, I realized that the miracle was not her survival, but God's undying love.

We are tempted to blame God or own own faithlessness, when the healing we want and miracle we yearn for fail to occur. As I pointed out in chapter four, health and illness are multidimensional. Further, as the apostle Paul asserts, our ability to discern the miraculous is limited: "we do not know how to pray as we ought" (Romans 8:26) and "we see in a mirror dimly" (1 Corinthians 13:12). Because of our limited vision, seldom do we fully know what is best for ourselves or others. Faithful agnosticism invites us to trust that God is working for the best in our lives even when it is not obvious to the superficial eye.

Prayer will not, for example, prevent aging but it may shape how we age. Spiritual centeredness enables us to face the necessary crises of life, knowing that whether we live or die, recover or live in infirmity, we are in God's hands. As I write these words, I am still marveling over a speech I heard by Cardinal Joseph Bernardin, one of America's most inspiring spiritual leaders. Faced with the prognosis of terminal illness, Cardinal Bernardin placed his trust in God and the resurrection faith. He was not cured, but he was surely healed!

As we consider the hope for miracles, it is important to remember that sound theology prevents us from false hope and false hopelessness. As I stated in the previous chapter, we need to avoid two sets of extremes in our quest to experience the power of prayer and the hope of the miraculous. First, we must avoid the extreme of omnipotence and impotence when we speak of God. God is not aloof or ineffectual, but God does not cause everything. God's aim is always toward beauty, healing, and love. God does not unilaterally or omnipotently determine the events of our lives, be they events of illness or healing. But, God works within the events of our lives to bring about the healing and well-being that is possible, given the particular situation as well as the global constellation of events. There are times, as the Scriptures suggest, when God's own desires are thwarted by human choice or natural disaster.

We must avoid the extremes of omnipotence and impotence

when speaking of our own spiritual powers or God's intervention in our lives. While our own spirituality contributes to our well-being, we do not fully determine our health and illness. One of the mysteries of life is the reality that saints die young and sinners die in their sleep after a long and prosperous life. Though we cannot fully "create our own reality" or bring miracles to pass by our own efforts, we are not victims either. Every spiritual state has physical correlates. We can make miracles possible by our own response to God's ever-present, creative love. We receive miracles when we: 1) open ourselves to God's presence in spiritual formation and whole person medical care, 2) participate as a receiver as well as giver in a vital and prayerful community of faith, 3) allow ourselves to take the risks of transformation that may call for death to the familiar so that new life may burst forth.

As we ponder the possibility of healing, we must take the widest temporal as well as geographical perspective. Our healing always takes place in the context of the multidimensional and infinitely dynamic body of Christ. As we look beyond the individual ego, moment, or lifetime toward the perspective of God, our image of healing is transformed. Indeed, there are times when death may not be the greatest evil, a temporary healing may not be the greatest good. We must not fear those things that kill the body, but those that kill the soul. Ultimately, the miracle we seek is to live and die in the presence and awareness of God. While we may not always be able to expect a miracle, we must depend upon the miracle of God's sustaining love that embraces those who recover as well as those who will never get well. The ultimate miracle is the "radical amazement" (Abraham Heschel) that we experience when we discover that "whether we live or die, we are with God."

Recently, I repainted my father's house. As I painted beside the plants and bushes, I was puzzled to find an array of weatherbeaten tennis balls, baseballs, and golf balls. Childhood memories of throwing the ball against the house flooded my mind. I had recovered the lost balls. My prayers had been answered from a broader perspective and according to a different timetable from the wishes of the child who once searched for lost balls in those very bushes. Now, the answer involved the undramatic repayment of my father's love by his now grown-up son.

Seen from the divine perspective, all of life is miraculous. The miracles we pray for and healings may already be here but our recognition of them comes on their own timetable and God's, and we must trust that in the grand ecology of the body of Christ, which is not limited by time or space, life or death, our deepest needs will be met. The miracle we need is right where we are, for by God's grace we are "the temple of God."

QUESTIONS FOR REFLECTION AND DISCUSSION

1) How do you define a miracle? Do miracles really occur?

2) How do you differentiate magic from miracle?

3) Do you think there are places or rituals that are more effective in bringing about miraculous experiences?

4) Do you think God can change the course of the universe? Do you think we can change God?

NOTES

Introduction

1. Herbert Benson, *The Relaxation Response* (New York: Avon, 1975) and *Beyond the Relaxation Response* (New York: Times Books, 1984).

2. Notable exceptions have been Morton Kelsey, *Psychology, Religion, and Christian Healing* (New York: Crossroad, 1988), Agnes Sanford, *The Healing Light* (St. Paul: Macalester Park Publishing, 1972), Francis MacNutt, *Healing* (Notre Dame: Ave Maria Press), and Bruce Epperly, *At the Edges of Life* (St. Louis: Chalice Press, 1992) and *Crystal and Cross* (Mystic, CT: Twenty-Third Publications, 1996).

Chapter 1

1. Larry Dossey, *Healing Words: The Power of Prayer and the Practice of Medicine* (San Francisco: HarperSan Francisco), 1994.

2. W.H. Auden, *For the Time Being: A Christmas Oratorio* in *Collected Poetry of W.H. Auden* (New York: Random House, 1945), p. 466.

Chapter 2

1. Quoted in Aldous Huxley, *The Doors of Perception* (New York: Harper and Brothers, 1954).

2. Dean Ornish's work is found in the following books: *Stress, Diet, and Your Health* (New York: Holt and Rinehart, 1982); *Dr. Dean Ornish's Program for Reversing Heart Disease* (New York: Random House, 1990); *Eat More, Weigh Less* (New York: HarperCollins, 1993). Each of these books contains extensive exercise, life-style, and dietary resources for persons seeking to transform their lives.

3. For example, Frances Lappe's *Diet for a Small Planet* (New York: Ballantine, 1984) or *Food First* (New York: Houghton Mifflin, 1977).

4. Andrew Weil, *Spontaneous Healing* (New York: Alfred A. Knopf, 1995).

5. Carole Perlmutter, "Natural Weight Control: Never Overeat Again," *Prevention* (September 1996).

6. Brother Lawrence, *Practice of the Presence of God* (Nashville: Upper Room, 1950).

7. Ronald Sider, *Rich Christians in an Age of Hunger: A Biblical Study* (Downers Grove: Intervarsity Press, 1980), p. 172.

8. Ibid., p. 182.

9. Plato, *Timaeus* (Indianapolis: Bobbs-Merrill, 1949), 87c, 88b.

10. Herbert Benson and Eileen Stuart, *The Wellness Book* (New York: Birch Lane Books, 1992), p. 121.

11. Julie Denison, "Not Less, But a Different Kind of Touch," *Christian Century* (February 21, 1991), pp. 200-203.

12. Ibid., p. 201.

13. Ibid., p. 201.

14. Dolores Krieger, *Therapeutic Touch* (Englewood Cliffs: Prentice-Hall, 1979).

15. W.H. Auden, *For the Time Being: A Christmas Oratorio* in *Collected Poetry of W.H. Auden* (New York: Random House, 1945), p. 466.

Chapter 3

1. Bernie Siegel, *Peace, Love, and Healing* (New York: Harper and Row, 1989), p. 18.

2. Louise Hay, *You Can Heal Your Life* (Santa Monica, CA: Hay House, 1984), p. 5.

3. Lawrence LeShan, *Cancer as a Turning Point* (New York: Penguin, 1994), p. 26.

4. Meyer Friedman and Roy Rosenman, *Type A Behavior and Your Heart* (New York: Alfred A. Knopf, 1975).

5. James Lynch, *The Language of the Heart* (New York: Basic Books, 1985) and *The Broken Heart* (New York: Basic Books, 1985).

6. O. Carl Simonton, Stephanie Matthews Simonton, and James Creighton, *Getting Well Again* (Los Angeles: J.P. Tarcher, 1978), p. 4.

7. Ibid., p. 10.

8. LeShan, *Cancer as a Turning Point*, p. 13.

9. Ibid., p. 111.

10. For an extended discussion of the role of hope and hopelessness in relationship to cancer see Lawrence LeShan, *You Can Fight for Your Life* (New York: M. Evans and Company, 1977).

11. Simonton, *Getting Well Again*, pp. 28-30.

12. Abraham Heschel, *The Sabbath* (New York: Farrar, Straus, and Giroux, 1988), p. 29.

13. Ibid., p. 18.

14. Tilden Edwards, *Sabbath Time* (New York: Seabury Press, 1982), p. 31.

15. Heschel, *The Sabbath*, p. 21.

16. One of the most helpful books on keeping the sabbath from a Christian perspective is Marva J. Dawn's *Keeping the Sabbath Holy* (Grand Rapids: Eerdmans, 1989).

17. Herbert Benson, *The Relaxation Response* (New York: Avon, 1975), pp. 74, 87-88.

18. Ibid., p. 74.

19. Herbert Benson, *Beyond the Relaxation Response* (New York: Times Books, 1984), p. 7.

20. Ibid., p. 8.

21. Ibid., p. 82.

22. Basil Pennington, *The Way Back Home* (New York: Paulist, 1969), p. 19.

23. Shad Helmstetter, *The Self-Talk Solution* (New York: William Morrow, 1987), p. 44.

24. Ibid., p. 53.

25. Ibid., p. 69.

26. Simonton, p. 78.

27. Dierdre Davis Brigham, *Imagery for Getting Well* (New York: William Norton, 1994), p. 16.

28. Belleruth Naperstek, *Staying Well with Guided Imagery* (New York: Warner Books, 1991), p. 20.

29. Simonton, p. 7.

30. David Fleming, S.J., *The Spiritual Exercises of St. Ignatius: A Literal Translation and a Contemporary Reading* (St. Louis: Institute of Jesuit Studies, 1978).

31. Ruth Carter Stapleton, *The Gift of Inner Healing* (Waco: Word Books, 1976), p. 10.

32. Ruth Carter Stapleton, *The Experience of Inner Healing* (Waco: Word Books, 1977), p. 10.

33. Ibid., p. 69.

34. Stapleton, *The Gift of Inner Healing*, p. 38.

Chapter 4

1. Larry Dossey, *Healing Words: The Practice of Prayer and the Power of Medicine* (San Francisco: HarperSanFrancisco, 1993), p. xv.

2. Ibid., pp. 179-86.

3. Dale Matthews; David Larson; Constance Berry, *The Faith Factor: An Annotated Bibliography of Clinical Research on Spiritual Subjects* (Rockville, MD: National Institute of Healthcare Research, 1993), I, 3.

4. Ibid., I, 11, 23.

5. Ibid., I, 25-26, 35.

6. Ibid., I, 53, 132.

7. Ibid., I, 46.

8. Marjorie Hewett Suchocki, *In God's Presence: Theological Reflections on Prayer* (St. Louis: Chalice Press, 1996), p. 5.

9. Ibid., p. 35.

10. Alfred North Whitehead, *Process and Reality: Corrected Edition* (New York: Free Press, 1978), p. 351.

11. The following books have been important in the lives of many spiritual seekers today: John Biersdorf, *The Healing of Purpose* (Nashville: Abingdon, 1985); Brother Lawrence, *The Practice of the Presence of God* (Nashville: Upper Room, 1950); Maxie Dunnam, *The Workbook of Intercessory Prayer* (Nashville: Upper Room, 1979), and *The Workbook of Living Prayer* (Nashville: Upper Room, 1974); Tilden

Edwards, *Living Simply Through the Day* (New York: Paulist, 1977); Richard Foster, *Prayer* (San Francisco: HarperSanFrancisco, 1992); Frank Laubach, *Prayer, the Mightiest Power in the World* (New York: Fleming Revell, 1946); Kenneth Leech, *True Prayer* (San Francisco: Harper and Row, 1986); Basil Pennington, *Centered Living* (Garden City: Doubleday, 1986).

12. Walter Wink, *Engaging the Powers* (Philadelphia: Fortress, 1992), p. 299.

Chapter 5

1. Bernie Siegel, *Love, Medicine, and Miracles* (New York: Harper and Row, 1986), p. 180.

2. Quoted in James Wagner, *Blessed to Be a Blessing* (Nashville: Upper Room, 1980), p. 35.

3. Francis MacNutt, *Healing* (Notre Dame: Ave Maria Press, 1974), p. 93.

4. Dan Wakefield, *Expect a Miracle* (San Francisco: HarperSanFrancisco, 1995), p. 6.

5. Ibid., p. 35.

6. Carolyn Miller, *Creating Miracles* (Tiburon, CA: J.P. Tarcher, 1992), p. 53.

7. Ibid., p. 57.

8. Ibid., p. 248.

9. Ruth Cranston, *The Miracle of Lourdes* (New York: McGraw-Hill, 1955), p. 94.

10. Ibid., p. 259.

11. Ibid., p. 271.

Of Related Interest...

Traits of a Healthy Spirituality
Melannie Svoboda, S.N.D.
This book is a great motivator for those developing their spiritual life. In an engaging style it defines and describes 20 indicators of a healthy spirituality such as self-esteem, joy, and commitment.
ISBN: 0-89622-698-0, 144 pp, $9.95 (order M-87)

Pursuing Wellness, Finding Spirituality
Richard Gilmartin
The author challenges today's men and women to develop life-styles that accept personal responsibility in order to nurture their own peace and happiness. This book holds the blueprint for the development of physical-psychological-spiritual well being.
ISBN: 0-89622-674-3, 208 pp, $12.95 (order M-62)

Get Real About Yourself
25 Ways to Grow Whole and Holy
William Larkin
The author encourages readers to improve their self-esteem as a means of developing a deeper relationship with God and others. Based in psychology, William Larkin's theories are colored with the elements of sound Christian living.
ISBN: 0-89622-606-9, 160 pp, $9.95 (order M-22)

Caring for Yourself When Caring for Others
Margot Hover
The author offers ways—including Scripture references, personal stories, and prayers—for caregivers to nourish and revitalize themselves. Filled with hope, humor, and experience as a caregiver, the author offers a very important series of reflections which should be required reading for anyone working as caregivers to others. The brief chapters address the big issues in this process.
ISBN: 0-89622-533-X, 88 pp, $7.95 (order C-91)

Available at religious bookstores or from:

TWENTY-THIRD PUBLICATIONS
P.O. Box 180 • Mystic, CT 06355

For a complete list of quality books and videos call:
1 - 8 0 0 - 3 2 1 - 0 4 1 1